Rapid Weight Loss Hypnosis for Woman

Extreme Weight Loss with Positive Affirmations, Meditation, and Hypnosis. Increase Your Self Esteem and Heal Your Body. Stop Food Addiction and Emotional Eating

Hypnosis Motivation Institute

Rapid Weight Loss Hypnosis for Woman
Written by: Hypnosis Motivation Institute

© Copyright 2020 - All rights reserved.

Table of Contents

INTRODUCTION 9

CHAPTER 1 – HYPNOSIS AND HYPNOTHERAPY 11

    What Is Hypnotherapy? 11

    What Is Hypnosis? 12

    Hypnosis Used For Entertainment 13

    How Does Hypnosis Work? 14

    How Does Hypnotherapy Work With Other Modalities? 15

    Who Can Be Hypnotized? 16

    Hypnosis For Weight Loss: The Golden Method Of Burning Fat Quickly And Permanently Through Hypnosis 17

    First, We Must Look At The Likely Causes Of This Programming. 18

    Healing The Body With Hypnosis 22

    Meditation Healing 24

    Meditation Techniques For Beginners 27

    Fat Burning With Activation With Hypnosis 30

    Amazing Things You Can Do With Hypnosis 34

    Hypnosis Is A Powerful Tool For Inner Transformation 34

    Hypnosis To Lose Weight - The Right Beginning For Quick Weight Loss .. 41

    Evidence That Hypnosis Is Useful 46

    Hypnosis And Hypnotherapy: Five Key Points 49

    Is Hypnosis Real? 51

CHAPTER 2 - HYPNOSIS WEIGHT LOSS SESSION 54

    Hypnosis For Weight Loss 54

Is Weight-Loss Hypnosis Effective? 56

How To Use Hypnosis To Change Eating Habits 61

Using Hypnosis In Different Ways 63

Hypnosis Is The Key To Your Mind And Your Health! 65

Guidelines For Suggestions: 68

CHAPTER 3 - A BASIC SELF-HYPNOSIS SESSION FOR WEIGHT LOSS 69

Self-Hypnosis: What It Is And What It Can Do 69

Hypnosis And Self Hypnosis For Weight Loss 72

Using Hypnosis For Weight Loss 73

How To Self-Hypnotize For Weight Loss 75

Self-Hypnosis For Weight Loss 80

CHAPTER 4 - HYPNOSIS PORTION CONTROL SESSION 85

Control And Start Eating The Right Amount 85

Why Is Portion Control Difficult? 87

These Tips For Managing Portions At Home: 91

CHAPTER 5 - GASTRIC BAND HYPNOTHERAPY 92

What Is A Gastric Band? 92

Gastric Band Hypnosis 93

Hypnotherapist Becca Teers Explains Why Diets Don't Work For Weight Loss: 94

The Benefits 94

What Are The Risks? 96

How Gastric Band Hypnosis Works 97

The Procedure 97

Will It Work For Me? 100

What Are The Advantages Of Gastric Band Hypnotherapy Over Surgery? 101

CHAPTER 6 - TIPS AND TRICKS FOR HYPNOSIS FOR WEIGHT LOSS 104

Weight Loss Hypnotists- Tips For Weight Loss 104

Top Ten Ways To Lose Weight 111

Weight Loss By Hypnosis- 7 Huge Benefits 120

CHAPTER 7 - BINGE EATING SUPPRESSION 127

Binge Eating 127

How To Know If Your Weight Is Suppressed 132

Binge Eating vs Overeating 133

5 Reasons People Binge Eat 134

How To Overcome Binge Eating 135

CHAPTER 8 - INSTRUCTIONS TO ENSURE THAT MEDITATION FOR WEIGHT LOSS 138

What Is Meditation? 138

What Are The Benefits Of Meditation For Weight Loss? 139

How Can I Start Meditating For Weight Loss? 141

Next, With Your Eyes Open Or Closed, Follow These Steps: 142

How Can Meditation Help You Lose Weight? 143

Where Can I Find Guided Meditations? 145

CHAPTER 9 - DEVELOPING A POSITIVE ATTITUDE WITH SELF-HYPNOSIS ... 147

Discover What Makes You Happy 147

Develop Positive Habits 148

Everyone Can Benefit 150

7 Positive Thinking Tips 151

CHAPTER 10 - WHAT IS INTUITIVE EATING? 154

The 4 Characteristics Of Intuitive Eating Are: 157

Steps To Becoming An Intuitive And Mindful Eater 161

8 Tips For Intuitive Eating 163

5 Intuitive Eating Mistakes You Don't Want To Make 165

Principles Of Intuitive Eating 170

Powerful Weight Loss Tip 174

CHAPTER 11 - BODY RESPECT 177

Here Are 10 Ways You Can Start Being Kind To Your Body And Give It The Respect It Deserves: 182

Here Are Ten Practical Tips On Using Body Language To Improve Your Life. 188

CHAPTER 12 - MEAL PLANNING 194

How To Meal Plan 194

A Meal Plan Diet Has Many Advantages: 196

Top Tips To Meal Planning For Weight Loss 200

What Is A Healthy Diet Meal Plan? 202

CHAPTER 13 - EMOTIONAL EATING 209

What Does Emotional Eating Mean? 209

4 Types Of Eating 210

How The Mood-Food-Weight Loss Cycle Works 216

How Do You Get Back On Track? 217

CHAPTER 14 - FASTING WEIGHT LOSS 227

Fast Weight Loss Strategies 228

7 Fast Weight Loss Tips To Speed Up Metabolism 229

Fast Weight Loss - Importance Of Boosting Metabolism 233

CONCLUSION 237

Introduction 240

Chapter 1: Hypnosis for Rapid Weight Loss 245

    How Hypnosis Works 246

    The Benefits of Hypnotherapy for Weight Loss 249

    Examples of Effective Hypnosis Sessions 251

    Step by Step: How You Will Lose Weight with Hypnosis 255

    Using Hypnosis to Encourage Healthy Eating and Discourage Unhealthy Eating 260

    Using Hypnosis to Encourage Healthy Lifestyle Changes 261

Chapter 2: Meditation to Burn Fat 264

    A Simple Daily Weight Loss Meditation 266

        The Meditation 267

    Fat Burning Meditation 271

        The Meditation 272

    A Deep Meditation for Weight Loss 277

        The Meditation 278

    Meditation for Cutting Calories 285

        The Meditation 286

    Strategies and Mind Exercises for Cutting Calories 288

        Affirmations 289

        Eating with the Right Mindset 289

        Short Meditations 290

        Eating Foods, You Enjoy 290

        Making Eating an Experience 291

        Mindful Eating 292

Chapter 3: Portion Control Hypnosis 293

Why Do People Overeat? 295

Getting to the Root Cause of Your Binge Eating 297

Learning to Avoid Temptations and Triggers 300

Tips for Managing Stress to Avoid Emotional Eating 302

Learning to Eat Intuitively 306

Getting Support When You Need It 310

Forgiving Yourself for Your Dietary Mistakes 314

Meditation for Portion Control 318

   The Meditation 319

Chapter 4: Affirmation to Cut Calories 323

What Are Affirmations, and How Do They Work? 323

How Do I Pick and Use Affirmations for Weight Loss? 326

What Should I Do with My Affirmations? 329

How Are Affirmations Going to Help Me Lose Weight? 331

Affirmations for Self-Control 333

Affirmations for Exercise 337

Affirmations for Healthier Habits 342

Affirmations for Self-Esteem 347

Affirmations for Beauty 352

A Guided Affirmation Meditation 357

   The Meditation 358

Chapter 5: Chakra Guided Meditation 364

What Are Your Chakras and How Do They Affect Weight Loss? ... 365

How Integrating Chakra Work Will Help You Lose Weight 371

The Seven Chakras and Their Nutritional Guides 376

Alternatives Ways to Relax and Nurture Your Chakras 382

A Guided Chakra Relaxation Meditation 390
    The Meditation 391
A Guided Chakra Meditation for Healing Your Body Image 397
    The Meditation 399
Conclusion 406

Part One

INTRODUCTION

The main advantage of gastric band hypnotherapy is that it allows a far more natural weight loss occurrence to take place. One thing all experts agree on is that drastic shifts in weight loss or weight gain are not good for the body and quite often with gastric band surgery, there is drastic weight loss.

Hypnosis is considered safe for most people if practiced under the guidance of a trained therapist. It isn't a means for brainwashing or mind control. Hypnosis can work by altering the way your mind responds to what your body is telling you, whether that's to exercise more, eating less by using a virtual gastric band or whatever it is you feel you need to do to lose weight.

While hypnosis may provide an edge over other weight loss methods, it isn't necessarily a quick fix. Still, hypnosis does suggest that using it in combination with nutritious food, daily exercise, and other therapies may help. A hypnotic gastric band is needed to evaluate the use of hypnosis for more significant weight loss. For extra support, consider asking your doctor for a referral to a nutritionist or other professional who may help you create an individual weight loss plan to reach your goals.

Intuitive eating is a nutrition philosophy that teaches people to become more attuned to the body's natural hunger and fullness signals to attain a healthy weight and to become a generally healthier person. It is a process that is intended to create a healthy relationship with food, mind, and body. Intuitive eating can also be called wise eating, conscious eating, non-diet approach, and normal eating.

Weight loss provides you with find easy-to-understand explanations and tips, tricks, and advice for quickly adapting Intuitive eating helps your needs in losing weight.

The idea is that you should eat when you're hungry and stop when you're full. It teaches you how to get in touch with your body cues like hunger, fullness, and satisfaction while learning to trust your body around food again.

Even if you have tried different diets or different kinds of stress management in the past and failed, this audiobook will help you get back in mental and physical shape with just a different commitment. The perspective of the problem is different, just change it and you will find the solution! Hypnosis and intuitive eating works in hand, has proven results in aiding weight loss.

CHAPTER 1 – HYPNOSIS AND HYPNOTHERAPY

Hypnosis And Hypnotherapy: What's The Difference?

What Is Hypnotherapy?

To understand the difference between hypnosis and hypnotherapy, think of hypnosis as a tool and hypnotherapy as the use of a tool. In SAT terms, hypnotherapy is to hypnotism as art therapy is to art.

The definition of hypnotherapy is clear from the word itself. Hypnotherapy is the practice of hypnosis for therapeutic purposes.

In other words, if you are a professional mental health therapist or medical doctor and you're using hypnosis to help a client overcome a mental or physical condition, you're practicing hypnotherapy.

The hypnotic trance state is a remarkably flexible tool for solving mental and physical health problems. Here are just a few ways mental health and medical professionals use hypnotherapy:

- ❖ Helping people quit smoking or reduce overeating by focusing their minds and suggesting healthier behavior.

- Accessing the mind-body link to relieve chronic and acute pain, including during surgery and childbirth. Hypnotherapy has also proven effective against stubborn physical afflictions like irritable bowel syndrome and dermatological conditions.
- Diving deep into the subconscious mind to uncover and treat the root causes of mental health issues such as depression, anxiety, PTSD, and addiction.
- We'll focus the rest of this article on that last use. As many hypnotherapists have discovered, the trance state is the key to unlocking the hidden depths of our minds, memories, and motivations.

What Is Hypnosis?

Hypnosis is the act of guiding someone into the trance state. Different experts define the trance state differently, but they almost always refer to:

- A deep state of relaxation.
- Hyperfocus and concentration.
- Increased suggestibility.

If that sounds commonplace, it's because it is. Most of us go in and out of the trance state regularly. If you've ever zoned out on your daily commute, fell into a reverie while listening to music, or found yourself immersed in the world of a book or movie, you've been in the trance state.

Hypnosis is often recognized as being used by performers in comedy or entertainment, and is typically seen as fun and harmless in those situations. However, hypnosis has broader applications when used in helping practices. Essentially, there are three main platforms for hypnosis:

The only difference between hypnosis and these everyday trance states is that, in hypnosis, someone induces the trance state to achieve something: healing, discovery, or stress relief, for example.

Hypnosis Used For Entertainment

Hypnosis used by a person trained in specialized uses, such as helping people to stop smoking, manage weight, or deal with sleeping problems.

Hypnosis used by a licensed mental health practitioner (hypnotherapist) as one of the tools in the counseling/therapeutic toolbox.

Hypnosis and hypnotherapy have an extensive history as reputable methods used the therapeutic process by trained and skilled hypnotists and hypnotherapists alike. The difference between hypnosis and hypnotherapy is that hypnosis is defined as a state of mind, while hypnotherapy is the name of the therapeutic modality in which hypnosis is used.

A trained hypnotist uses hypnosis to help people with issues such as smoking cessation and weight management but is not licensed to practice hypnotherapy. Hypnotherapy is practiced by a hypnotherapist who is a trained, licensed, and/or certified professional. Only a hypnotherapist may use hypnotherapy to work with such mental health concerns as phobias, stage fright, eating disorders, and certain medical conditions.

How Does Hypnosis Work?

Hypnosis is defined as a harmless altered trance state characterized by very deep relaxation, highly focused attention, and an extreme openness to suggestions that are usually positive and foster positive therapeutic changes. However, a hypnotic trance is not necessarily therapeutic on its own. For example, when someone is driving to the mall, seemingly suddenly arrives, and is not sure exactly how he or she got there so soon, he/she has experienced an altered, hypnotic state. People may also experience this altered state when they are just beginning to fall asleep and are in a dreamy and drowsy state, aware but not completely focused—just focused enough to have a simple conversation but not remember talking at all.

When used for therapeutic approaches, specific suggestions and images given to people in a trance can positively alter their behavior. When in this state of hypnosis, you are more inclined to permanent change and more likely to be successful in making the lasting changes you desire. Almost all lasting changes happen in your subconscious mind.

Another example of how visualization in hypnosis works is when a hypnotherapist helps a person experiencing claustrophobia to visualize being in a very open space, without fear, when entering an elevator. By learning to positively visualize entering the elevator without fear, the person is often able to then do it in reality. The subconscious mind does not distinguish between a genuine experience and a suggested one. If you visualize it in a trance state, your body will react to it.

How Does Hypnotherapy Work With Other Modalities?

"Learning hypnotherapy does not commit you to drastically changing your therapy practice," says hypnotherapist Catherine Reiss. "The training will allow you to more quickly and effectively get to the cause of your clients' unwanted behaviors and the feelings they present with it, but it also facilitates the use of trance in more traditional formats."

Once hypnotherapy has opened up the door to your clients' repressed memories and emotions foregoing months or years of arduous talk therapy you can set yourself to the task of healing using your tried-and-true techniques.

"One can continue to do cognitive behavioral therapy and add the use of trance and hypnotherapy techniques," Reiss says.

Cognitive-behavioral therapy (CBT), in particular, is an effective complement to hypnotherapy.

Who Can Be Hypnotized?

The simplest answer is that almost anyone can be hypnotized if they want to be. Modern research has shown that most people can be hypnotized to some degree and that the real question is how deep and to what degree they go into trance. Being able to be hypnotized is not a sign of being weak-minded, gullible, or giving up control. The ability to be hypnotized—or "hypnotizability"—is correlated with intelligence and the ability to have heightened awareness and focus while being in complete control.

For example, if while in a hypnotic trance you were asked to give the hypnotherapist your wallet or take off all of your clothes, you wouldn't unless you truly wanted to. Likewise, if you were in the audience of a stage performance by a hypnotist and you were selected to participate in the show, you would quack like a duck only if you truly wanted to. The participants are usually chosen because the hypnotist believes you want to act silly and be part of the show. This is in contrast to someone who is not showing any indication he or she wants to be at the event or even have fun.

Hypnosis For Weight Loss: The Golden Method Of Burning Fat Quickly And Permanently Through Hypnosis

If you are overweight you may be tired of everyone telling you that losing weight is just about eating less food and or consuming fewer calories. You may have tried every diet old and new. But, sometimes it seems that our bodies have found a way to turn a plate of lettuce into a pound of fat! Many people who attempt weight loss discover sooner or later their efforts are complicated by metabolic programming that keeps weight on the body regardless of how one changes their eating habits. If you or your friend or client is overweight and you'd like to see if such programming is affecting weight loss efforts take the following questionnaire:

- ❖ Do you find that no matter how much you starve yourself the
- ❖ Weight just doesn't fall off as quickly as it should?
- ❖ Do you find yourself eating less than your more slender
- ❖ Friends and still don't lose weight?
- ❖ Do you find your food cravings going way up even as the

- Pounds begin to fall off? As if you were starving instead of dieting?
- Do you become tired and lethargic when dieting?
- Do you gain back all the weight you've lost from a diet with alarming speed?

If you answered "yes" to any of these questions you probably have some subconscious metabolic programming to hold weight on your body instead of burning it up for energy as it should. Now here's the good news! There are many ways we can deal with this programming through hypnosis so you don't have to fight your body as well as your food cravings to lose weight!

First, We Must Look At The Likely Causes Of This Programming.

The metabolism of food is the intricate process by which nutrients from food are consumed and utilized by the body. It is a complex process in which several factors are involved. One is the function of the thyroid gland, the "master switch" which regulates the rate of cellular metabolism. Through hypnotic imagery, we can turn up the production of thyroxin, the primary metabolic hormone produced by the thyroid gland.

More thyroxin means more fat burned more weight loss and more energy for you. There may be medical reasons for thyroid dysfunction, which is why we suggest a full physical examination and possible testing of your thyroid function before proceeding with a course of hypnotherapy.

Another key element to the body's metabolic processes is the activity of two key pancreatic hormones: insulin and glucagons. These key metabolic hormones cause our body to store or burn fat. The types of food you eat directly affect the activities of these hormones. In general, it seems that most carbohydrates, including sugars, cause the secretion of insulin, which increases sugar metabolism and storage. Glucagons, secreted after a low carb meal, help the body burn protein and d fat, including the body's fat reserves.

This is part of the reason low carb diets are becoming popular. So how does hypnosis help you change your eating choices? Because all eating habits become rooted in the subconscious mind, simply deciding to eat differently rarely is sufficient to create long term changes in our eating habits. The imagery of hypnosis targets these subconscious programs and changes them in a way that is both permanent and nearly effortless. Personal hypnotic scripts which can be recorded on a self-hypnosis tape and listened to every night in bed can be created by working with a Hypnotherapist. Besides, it is of critical importance to address emotional eating habits.

Exercise is also a key component in the activation of metabolism. Researchers have discovered that regular exercise, even as little as thirty minutes a day, speeds up metabolism not only during exercise but also for many hours afterward, even when you are resting. Of course, many of us have a hard time with exercise. Enter again the power of hypnosis. Hypnotic suggestions can be used to increase one's motivation toward physical activity as well as increase strength and endurance. But often it takes much more than direct hypnotic suggestion to get more involved with exercise again.

One of the innovative processes we use can take you back to what you enjoyed doing physically as a child. You can pick one or two of these activities that you will again enjoy! We use the power of hypnosis to bring back the excitement you experienced as a child at play. We can also return to those traumatic experiences that caused us to turn ourselves off to the joys of physical activity, and rescue the past self from these traumas. An experience of being rejected, humiliated or injured on the playground in a team sport, for example, can lead one to shut down the desire to play outside. Our rescue mission allows the child to receive comfort and a promise of safety from the adult self along with an invitation to play outside in a new way with the adult.

One of the more common sources of metabolic programming is genetic. Some human genetic lines (South

Pacific Islander and Eskimos provide just two extreme examples) preserve fat on their bodies more readily because these traits served their ancestors well for thousands of years, especially in times of

famine. Changing these genetic codes within our DNA may be difficult for even the most skilled practitioners. However, with hypnosis, we can persuade the metabolism to override these DNA programs and help us let go of fat. Many times my clients have said to me "My whole family is overweight!" This is the time to utilize specific hypnotic suggestions geared to override DNA programming.

Another common theme among those who struggle with weight loss is that the subconscious mind may be afraid to lose weight because if one's weight problems disappear than one might have to face other scarier issues. One client told me in trance that if she lost that weight over which she was obsessing she would have to "Do something with my life, and I don't know what to do!" At the Institute we can test for these issues and offer a plan of healing. One valuable technique that can be used here is a journey to the future self to discover how to successfully fulfill one's life purpose.

Another common theme I have discovered among women clients with metabolic programming to stay fat is the body's need to insulate itself with fat to protect itself from unwanted sexual advances. A large number of obese clients are victims of childhood sexual abuse. Many others have gained weight to silence their own unmet sexual needs within an unfulfilling marriage. Others use weight as an excuse not to meet men and thus risk rejection or betrayal. If you are not aware of such subconscious programming it could be deeply buried in the subconscious mind, and still, be affecting your metabolism. Your hypnotherapist can help you discover and heal these problems. I have personally experienced great success in rescuing clients from early sexual abuse trauma, which has often resulted in rapid weight loss without any apparent dietary change.

Healing The Body With Hypnosis

How To Heal Yourself

You can learn how to heal yourself! You are the only one who can. The right food, the right exercise, the right medications, the right relationships -all these can help support your healing process, but not unless you intentionally cause them to. Your conscious, intentional mind (which is separate from, though connected to, your subconscious mind and nervous system) is the key to your self-healing.

The Process Is Simple

- ❖ First, you need to understand the process with your intellect, the part capable of critical thinking that realizes the value of evidence-based reasoning.

- ❖ The next step in healing any system is that the system becomes aware of its identity as a system. For you, this means freeing yourself from distraction and focusing on who you are, your true values, purpose, goals, and vision.

- ❖ Third, you learn how to read the signals and messages that come from within and how to balance your system physically, mentally, and emotionally.

Fortunately, you can learn to do this in a remarkably short period using the powerful Mind Tools These tools can help you to reach a very pleasant state of deep relaxation and meditation, bringing you into the present, emptying your mind of distractions and your body of toxins, and preparing the cells of your body to receive your self-healing instructions.

Another very valuable tool for self-healing is guided imagery. This process involves holding specific healing imagery in the mind while in the receptive "Healing State." This results in relief of stress, and the activation of your unconscious healing and corrective processes are mobilized. You are "reprogramming" your mind and rewiring your brain. Your goal is to restore internal coherence and balance, and thus to help heal your body, emotions, mind, and behavior.

People struggling with chronic pain or other medical conditions can use healing meditation to feel better in body and spirit. Some report dramatic results from healing meditation, while others simply appreciate the reduction in stress that comes from sitting quietly and focusing the mind. Healing meditation often incorporates visualization techniques.

Meditation Healing

What To Expect

While meditation hasn't been proven to cure specific ailments, patients report that it can be helpful when used alongside more conventional treatments. Meditation can help reduce anxiety, for one thing, which can potentially cause positive changes in your body. It's important to be open to the process and have faith that it will help, but be willing to give it time.

Guided Meditation Techniques

Guided imagery, in which you create mental pictures in response to another person's instructions, is commonly used for healing meditation. For example, if you have cancer, you might be asked to vividly picture your white blood cells fighting and winning against the cancer cells, and purging the bad cells from your body.

Personal Healing Images

You can use a healing meditation CD, or you can develop your powerful healing images. For example, you might visualize your immune system as a train chugging steadily up a hill. Try to meditate on your chosen image often, at least once a day. You can also turn to it whenever you need a mental boost.

Preparing For Healing Meditation

When learning how to meditate, beginners often have trouble finding the best posture for meditation. Don't be afraid to experiment — there's no "right" way to meditate. Prepare to meditate by finding a quiet room without disruptions and take the following steps:

Turn Off Your Phone And Any Other Gadgets.

Dim The Lights

Sit in a straight-backed chair with your head forward, knees bent at a right angle and your hands on your thighs. You can also sit with your legs crossed or, if you're flexible, pretzel your legs into a lotus position. If sitting isn't comfortable, lie on the floor (it's too easy to fall asleep on a bed).

You can chant a mantra to yourself, such as " Om Mani Padme Hum," a Tibetan healing mantra, or use a simple word like "calm," "one" or "om."

Close Your Eyes Or Try Staring At A Focal Point

The best advice for beginners just learning about meditation is to start simple. Quieting your mind for long periods is more difficult than it looks, so just carve out 10 to 20 minutes a day at first. All you'll need is a quiet space where you won't be disturbed.

Benefits Of Meditation

Regular meditation can help relieve stress, improve your ability to focus and lead to a better understanding of your thought patterns and processes. Some people use meditation to enhance creativity, reduce chronic pain, treat headaches and even improve athletic performance.

Focus

Although most people meditate with closed eyes, many beginners find it useful to have a point of focus, such as a candle. Concentrating on the flame can make it easier to clear your mind.

When learning how to meditate, beginners tend to get frustrated by the persistence of outside thoughts all the anxieties, to-do lists and random memories that parade constantly through the brain. Instead of fighting them off, simply observe them as they enter your mind and let them pass. Repeating a mantra to yourself is another good way to maintain your focus.

Meditation Techniques For Beginners

Breathing meditation and relaxation meditation methods are especially good for people first learning to meditate. With breathing meditation, you simply breathe deeply from your abdomen, focusing all your attention on your breath, inhaling slowly through your nose and exhaling through your mouth. Relaxation meditation involves consciously visualizing the release of tension from your body, beginning at the head and moving slowly down to the toes.

Meditate In Action

"Walking meditation" is another useful way for beginners to learn how to meditate. The key is to concentrate fully on each deliberate step, paying attention only to the present moment. Focus on the rhythmic motion of your legs and the feel of the ground under your feet. Other active forms of meditation include tai chi and qigong (both traditional Chinese movement therapies) and yoga.

Combine Meditation With Lifestyle Choices

A healthy diet, regular exercise, and good sleep all enhance the positive effects of meditating. Spending time in nature, getting out in the sunshine, spending time with loved ones and trying to maintain a good attitude should also improve your results.

Healing The Body - How Listening To The Body Can Help You

Hypnosis is a powerful modality that can literally help your body to stop unwanted habits and then start healing and rejuvenating the body. It's all about the computer system that is located within the brain. The main purpose of hypnosis is to help you understand and gain control over your emotions or to help you improve your body's functioning, including your immune system. When you are hypnotized, you are open to suggestions and this can be used to help improve mind, body, spirit and immune system. What is your body telling you about the need for healing the body in your own life? The body sends out signals each day that let you know how healthy in general it is. Aches and pains are generally a sign that something is amiss somewhere deep inside. Some of the sources are a little more obvious than others. It is up to you to take the time to listen to the cues your body is providing about your overall health.

Positive Thinking

Almost every religion in the world mentions the important role positive thinking plays in healing. When healing the body becomes a priority for you, it is a good idea to spend a little time each day thinking positively. You just might find you have made a believer in this ages-old philosophy out of yourself in no time as you begin to feel the power of positive thinking working within your on body creating a healthy you.

Exercise

One of the most overlooked factors in healing the body is exercise. It has been relegated to a fitness role over the years and equated with the need for staying in shape or to aid in that pursuit rather than a healthy activity in and of itself. Exercise releases endorphins that provide relief from pain and an overall sense of happiness and well being.

Healthy Diet

As much as it may pain you to realize, a healthy diet is a great tool for healing the body. You need certain nutrients to retain optimal health. Unfortunately, we live in a fast-food world and very few people get the nutrients necessary for optimal health. For this reason, it is important to keep other options in mind such as vitamin supplements -although they aren't nearly as effective as getting the nutrients through your diet.

Adopt Healthy Habits

There are certain behaviors you can adopt that will promote better health. Replace your regular hand soap with antibacterial soap. Wash your hands often and wash them well. Teach your family to wash hands, cover mouths, and use sanitizing hand wipes or liquid cleaners in public to lower the risk of bringing infections and illnesses home. These habits may seem overly simplistic but they can result in helping heal the body through prevention, which is always the best cure.

Healing The Body With Hypnosis

Self-hypnosis is yet another way to heal the body from all manner of illnesses. Whether you are trying to reject cancer that is trying just as hard to take over or warding off the common cold many ways mastering the art of self-hypnosis can aid in your struggle. Hypnosis can help you relax, open your mind to positive thinking, help you allow the nutrients to go where they will be served best, and aid in boosting immunity among other great things.

Take Control Of Your Healing Process

It's time for you to retake control of your body and its healing process. Whether you use one or all of the techniques above you can find real aid when it comes to healing the body if you listen to your body and react accordingly - for the best possible health outcome.

Fat Burning With Activation With Hypnosis

Fat Busting Tips

If you want to shed a few extra pounds then these 9 tips will help you to lose weight and become thinner. Remember that easy weight loss is possible and that you can become the shape and size you want through consistent focus.

Tip 1: Fresh Fruits And Vegetables

The modern Western diet is one of the fatty processed foods with fresh fruit and vegetables pretty much sidelined (or at least processed with sugar added to them). Eating more fresh fruit and vegetables helps you not only to lose weight but boosts your energy, reduces your calorie intake, and provides you with a whole host of vital vitamins, minerals, and antioxidants that will help keep your body looking young and feeling fantastic.

Tip 2 : Eat More Often, But Eat Smaller Meals

Rather than eating the usual two big meals each day and then feeling like a sloth afterward, try eating more meals of smaller portions. If you eat about six or seven small meals at two or three-hour intervals, it keeps your metabolism and energy levels high, helping you to lose weight.

Tip 3: No Overeating And No Starving

Most people who diet yoyo between not eating and overeating. This confuses your body because when you overeat your body stores fat and when you starve yourself your body stores fat (it thinks there is a famine happening). Successful dieters still keep on eating, but carefully select WHAT they eat.

Tip 4 : No Skipping Breakfast

Yes, I know it's tempting, you're busy, you want an extra five minutes in bed, but don't skip breakfast. A good healthy breakfast stops you from overeating and studies show it controls your appetite and blood sugar levels throughout the day. Avoid

Tip 5 : Exercise

It's a dirty word I know, but it's a vital part of any weight loss program. Many people try to just reduce their calorie intake and not increase their level of physical activity. They then wonder why they are not losing any weight. Combine a reduced-calorie diet with an increased level of physical activity and you are virtually guaranteed to lose weight. Do 20-30 minutes of physical exercise (which does include walking) every day.

Tip 6: Drink Lots Of Water

When you go on a diet you tend to reach for diet drinks. They still hold calories and all sorts of other chemicals that get in the way of your weight loss program. Instead of drinking sugary or carbonated drinks, drink plenty of water. Around 8-10 glasses of water, a day helps to detox your body and has absolutely no calories in at all.

Tip 7 : Remove Toxins From Your Body

With the number of processed foods we all eat, toxins build up in our bodies. A simple way to remove them (and very cheap) is to fill a large flask with boiling water in the morning and squeeze the juice of one lemon into it. Then every half an hour drink a small amount of this. You'll find your tongue feels furry after the first day but after just 2-3 days you will be feeling great as the toxins come out of your system.

Tip 8: Don't Eat Too Late

With a hectic lifestyle, many people eat their main meal late at night. The trouble is the human body doesn't like eating late at night. When you eat after about 8 pm, you do not properly digest the meal you've eaten. The food tends to sit in your stomach and you are more inclined to convert it to fat. Try eating a light meal in the evening and your main meal earlier in the day.

Tip 9 : Keep On Moving

Our modern culture is one where we spend our lives sitting in front of a computer or television. We are incredibly sedentary. Humans are not designed for this type of lifestyle and so food eaten tends to get converted into fat. Burn excess fat by keep on moving. Fidget, exercise, walk around. This will help you burn extra calories.

Just by following these 9 steps, you can lose weight easily and permanently!

Amazing Things You Can Do With Hypnosis

By now you should have a good idea of what hypnosis is and what hypnosis is not. Now I want to show you what you, as a hypnotist, can do with hypnosis. After all, what is the point of being able to hypnotize someone if you do not know what you can do with them after you have them in hypnosis?

Also, if you are the one being hypnotized, you will discover many of the amazing things that hypnosis can do for you. After you read this post, you will know what your options are and what you can look forward to! , With that said, let us go ahead and take a look at what hypnosis is capable of.

Hypnosis Is A Powerful Tool For Inner Transformation

To start with, it is important to realize that our beliefs, feelings, and behaviors originate from within us at an unconscious level, and those very things are what determine our experience of reality, whether it be pleasant or unpleasant. Oftentimes we want to change those beliefs, feelings, and behaviors that cause our experience of reality to be unpleasant or do not produce the results we desire. Herein lies a problem. Most of our attempts at change seem to be short-lived and fruitless. It can seem so difficult to make the changes we desire as if we are always going uphill. The reason for this is that we attempt to make changes on a conscious level using willpower and whatever motivation we can muster up. When our willpower runs low or our motivation drops off, we find ourselves back at square one. Sound familiar?

The thing is, to truly make those changes you desire, you must make them at a subconscious level for the changes to be effective and permanent. Also, when you make those changes on a subconscious level, you will find that it is a whole lot easier than the will power/temporary motivation method. You may be wondering, "But how do I make changes from the inside out?" Well, that is where hypnosis comes into the picture. You see, hypnosis is like a bridge to your subconscious mind that allows you to gain access to parts of yourself to which you do not normally have access. Hypnosis allows you to learn new ways of believing, thinking, feeling, and behaving at a subconscious level. This is fantastic because all true learning happens at a subconscious level!

Now Let Us Take A Look At Some Of The Amazing Things That Hypnosis Can Do.

1. You Can Control Your Physiology Using Hypnosis.

Did you know that it can be healthy to go into hypnosis? Studies show that your immune system gets stronger under hypnosis. As I said before, hypnosis is like a bridge to your subconscious mind, and because your subconscious mind controls your physiology, through hypnosis you can change things like:

- Heartbeat/pulse rate
- Blood sugar
- Body temperature
- Metabolism
- Bleeding
- Breathing rate

2. You Can Manage Pain With Hypnosis.

Hypnosis has been used for years to manage and relieve pain. Studies have revealed that hypnosis works by decreasing the brain's response to pain signals and also helps deal with the psychological part of the pain that can make pain seem even more intense. People have used hypnosis to control pain in situations like:

- Car accidents (while waiting for help to arrive)
- Giving birth/hypnobirthing
- Managing chronic pain
- Undergoing major surgeries
- Relieving headaches
- Having cancer treatment

3. Health Problems Can Be Alleviated Using Hypnosis.

Many health problems are brought about by psychological causes. It is no secret that the way we think, feel, and believe can have a direct effect on our health. Ever heard of psychosomatic illnesses? Additionally, some behaviors result from psychological imbalances that can harm our health, such as drug use, smoking, overeating, and lack of exercise to name a few. Finally, there are genuine physical causes that are the root of some illnesses.

Thankfully, hypnosis can help deal with each of the areas mentioned above. Here are a few areas where hypnosis has been used successfully to alleviate health problems:

- Insomnia
- Skin conditions
- Obesity/weight control
- Allergies
- Anorexia/bulimia
- Asthma
- High blood pressure
- Irritable bowel syndrome
- Impotence
- Many more

4. You Can Heal Emotional Problems With Hypnosis.

As I am sure you are aware, the way you believe and think at a subconscious level will have a direct effect on how you feel. Also, how you feel has a lot to do with how much you enjoy life and how you behave. The way you currently believe and think was mostly conditioned into you at a young age and has been absorbed subconsciously. Hypnosis can be used to find the causes behind the way you feel, to "un-learn" those old ways of believing and thinking, and learn new, healthier, and more empowering ways to believe and think. Here is just a very short list of emotional problems that can be treated effectively with hypnosis:

- ❖ Anxiety/stress/nervousness
- ❖ Depression
- ❖ Self-esteem/confidence issues
- ❖ Anger
- ❖ Guilt
- ❖ Fears and phobias
- ❖ And the list goes on

5. You Can Gain Freedom From Addictions And Bad Habits With Hypnosis.

Listen, I am not a psychologist. However, from what I do know of psychology and from personal experience, addictive behaviors and bad habits seem to be a result of the emotional imbalances mentioned above as well as the ways of thinking and believing that are at the root of those imbalances. Let me be clear, that is an over-simplification of what is behind addictive behaviors and bad habits. I am just trying to break these ideas down so they can be easily understood.

Now, in the same way, that hypnosis can help a person deal with the emotional problems mentioned above, it can also help deal with the addictive behaviors and bad habits that result from them. Let us list a few addictive behaviors and bad habits that hypnosis can help a person gain freedom from:

Examples Of Addictive Behaviors

- Smoking
- Alcohol
- Cutting
- Drugs
- Sex/porn/masturbation
- Shopping
- Internet
- Gaming
- Gambling
- And many, many more
- Examples of bad habits
- Nail-biting
- Bed-wetting
- Lying

- Stealing/kleptomania
- Impulsive spending
- Selfishness
- Negative thinking
- Procrastination
- And many, many more

6. Hypnosis Can Improve The Overall Quality Of Your Life.

All right! Now, with all emotional problems healed and with those addictive behaviors and bad habits dealt with, now what? Well, you do not want to take something away without replacing it with something better, or at least of equal value. Just as hypnosis can help you "un-learn" those old ways of believing, thinking, feeling, and behaving, it can help you turn right around and "re-learn" new and better ways of believing, thinking, feeling, and behaving. Here are a few examples of how your life can improve with hypnosis:

- Motivation to exercise
- Healthier eating habits
- Increased fulfillment in relationships
- Emotional well-being/happiness
- Better sex!
- Increased health
- More positive mental outlook
- Confidence/improved self-esteem
- And much, much more!

Hypnosis To Lose Weight - The Right Beginning For Quick Weight Loss

If you are looking for the answer to quick weight loss then the steps I'm about to reveal to you will be the solution to your weight loss problems. Read carefully the steps that I am about to outline for your success with hypnosis to lose weight. The following outline of behavioral changes will accelerate your weight loss and when you combine them with a self-hypnosis program you will have successfully integrated a lifestyle change in your life that will guarantee your success at getting to your ideal weight.

Get Moving

Start some kind of activity. If you have a pedometer that measures the number of steps you take, wear it all day to keep track of your daily steps. 10,000 steps are what your goal is. This is minimal. You can add in some race walking for 30 minutes if you haven't reached your step count during your normal daily activities.

Eat Healthier Whole Foods

Eat fresh fruits and vegetables. 5 servings of fresh vegetables and 4 servings of fresh fruits each day. Select your fresh fruits and vegetables at each meal before you add in your healthy protein. This is the cornerstone of a healthier meal plan. You will also fill up quickly and have less room for unhealthy foods. More fiber means healthier elimination of toxins and fat. Hey- it's got to leave your body somehow! And that's what we want.

Get Out The Sugar

Eliminate sugar and sugar replacements, except for stevia. There is nothing nutritionally necessary in sugar or sugar substitutes, so get rid of them. Get your sweetness naturally from the fresh fruits you'll be eating more of. When you think sweet - think fresh fruit. Stop drinking sodas, pop, or canned or pre-bottled juices and juice drinks. Start drinking water. Clean, refreshing, cleansing water. Green tea is a good alternative to coffee or soda. It has also been shown to increase metabolism and it has some other healthy properties. You don't need specific weight loss green tea, just choose a good tasting green tea, brew it yourself. It's pretty easy to just boil water and steep a tea bag for a couple of minutes.

Cut Down On Fats

Reduce the fats that you eat. Stop eating anything with hydrogenated fats and reduce the other fats you consume. Eliminate fried foods. Take a fish oil supplement to make sure you get the right amount of essential oils in your diet.

Eliminate Diet Foods

Stop buying and eating any low fat or no-fat foods. These are not nourishing your body at all and deprive your body of the essentials of health. The original and only diet food you need is pure, whole foods. Whole fresh fruits and fresh vegetables. If this new plan is unfamiliar to you then you can help ease into this program with self-hypnosis to lose weight. Hypnosis is the best way to use mental rehearsal to quickly become familiar with new behaviors and introduce them into your lifestyle for fast results.

Fast Weight Loss Is Easy With Hypnosis

It is widely accepted that you must work on the mental and emotional aspects to lose weight. No one wants to count calories, measure, portions, kill themselves with grueling exercise, crave, binge, feel deprived, eat food that they dislike or suffer a starvation diet that has them feeling hungry and miserable. Everyone who wants to reduce in size wants fast weight loss.

The problem with the current popular programs is that they only work on what is going on below the neck. Hypnosis focuses on what is happening above the neck and in your head. Fast weight loss can be programmed into the subconscious mind so that everyday activities such as sitting at a desk, talking on the telephone or the very action of picking up the phone, will cause your body to respond by losing weight, and continue to lose until you reach your desired goal.

Many prominent publications such as Journals Of Consulting and Clinical Psychology have numerous studies regarding the efficiency of hypnosis on losing weight. As an example, a study of fifty females showed fast weight loss with hypnosis in comparison to the control group, which experienced much lower success. The American Medical Association approved hypnosis in 1958. As of then, it is being used adequately for various reasons such as pain management, smoking cessation, self-improvement, and sports training.

It is documented that with the proper suggestions; people can experience fast weight loss. Hypnosis creates a state of awareness to help people learn to look at food differently, to change eating habits and reduce cravings. More and more people are starting to see hypnosis as a solution because it makes losing weight fun and easy. Are you ready to learn the true secret to fast weight loss? Quit eating junk food. That is correct. The chemicals that cause weight gain and make it impossible to lose weight are in junk food. High fructose corn syrup is the biggest problem. Want to shrink in size? Stop eating junk food.

Hypnosis is a scientific preferred method of losing weight because it is safe, natural and effective. This process is simple because your mind is programmed to think differently about food. Most people don't have the discipline or self-control to stay committed to a plan that is hard and difficult. You can experience fast weight loss with hypnosis. This process creates a mind and body connection that will allow you to gain control of your eating habits and lose weight. The real secret to your success is properly programming the subconscious mind. While in hypnosis a person can be suggested that food is less important to them. Suggestions can also be given so that you can experience fast weight loss. Just like magic, it can be fast, easy and exciting. When food is less important, it is also less controlling. Hypnosis can help you stop thinking about food, therefore you eat less and lose weight.

If you want to close the door on improper eating habits and eliminate bad foods, hypnosis can provide the answer. Hypnosis can be used to help overcome emotional eating. Do you know what it would be like to be disappointed about missing an exercise session? Proper programming cannot only cause you to experience fast weight loss but also motivate you to love to exercise. Reducing stress and sleeping better are two additional positive benefits to the hypnosis process. If you want to be happier, calmer, thinner, and get off the diet roller coaster, hypnosis is the ticket for you. Sit back and watch your waistline shrink down to its proper size.

Evidence That Hypnosis Is Useful

Well, that depends on what you want to use it for. This article will help you cut through the marketing hype and find out what the scientific evidence is for the effectiveness of the most commonly sought-out hypnosis treatments. The information in this article is based on a review of current mainstream scientific research.

Is Weight Loss Hypnosis Effective? Yes, Hypnotherapy Does Help Long-Term Sustained Weight Loss.

The study "Hypnotic Enhancement of Cognitive-Behavioral Weight Loss Treatments" investigated the effectiveness of adding weight loss hypnosis to cognitive-behavioral treatments. The study concluded that hypnosis improves the effectiveness of a weight loss program.

Does Hypnosis Help Quitting Smoking? Yes, Hypnotherapy Does Help Long-Term Success In Quitting Smoking.

There have been many scientific studies conducted to investigate the effectiveness of smoking hypnosis. The evidence is positive that it does help people quit smoking. In 2007, Science Daily published a study that determined that hospital patients who were given hypnosis sessions for quitting smoking were more likely to quit smoking than people who used other methods. Dr. Faysal Hasan, who conducted the study, said: "hypnotherapy appears to be quite effective and a good modality to incorporate into a smoking cessation program after hospital discharge." The study included the use of self-hypnosis tapes as part of the follow-on treatment.

Is Relaxation Hypnosis Effective? Yes, Hypnotherapy Does Help With Increasing Relaxation.

Several scientific studies have investigated relaxation hypnosis, and have found it to be effective.

In summary, the British Medical Journal's article "Does Hypnosis Work for Relaxation?" states that there is good evidence that hypnosis can help promote relaxation and reduce anxiety.

Can Hypnotherapy Be Used To Treat Depression? Maybe, But More Research Is Needed.

In a 1998 study published in the Archives of General Psychiatry to research the effectiveness of complementary therapies for depression, researchers found no conclusive evidence that hypnotherapy helps with depression. Those researchers did note that there was limited evidence that relaxation therapies (which include hypnosis) can help with depression, but more research is needed for conclusive results.

Does Hypnosis Work For Anxiety? Yes, Hypnotherapy Significantly Reduces Anxiety And Can Reduce The Need For Anxiety-Related Medications.

How Can Hypnosis Benefit Cancer Patients? Hypnotherapy helps with pain management and reducing chemotherapy side effects. There have been many studies designed to address the use of hypnosis with cancer patients. Most of these studies have addressed pain management and reducing the adverse side effects of chemotherapy. The evidence is overwhelmingly positive.

Can Hypnosis Treat Irritable Bowel Syndrome? Yes, Hypnotherapy Is Highly Effective For Treating Irritable Bowel Syndrome.

The International Journal of Gastroenterology and Hepatology, GUT, has reported that in patients under 50 hypnosis can have a 100% success rate in treating irritable bowel syndrome. Self-hypnosis has been proven to be very effective for many physical and psychological conditions. Before choosing a hypnotherapist or self-hypnosis program, make sure that the person or product has a track record of success for the things you want to change in your life.

Hypnosis And Hypnotherapy: Five Key Points

Hypnosis Can Help With A Variety Of Problems

In a nutshell, Hypnosis can be used for anything which involves changing an existing mindset. Impatient people can learn to be more fore bearing through hypnosis; people who tend to gossip can tame their wagging tongue. Many people use self-hypnosis to improve their grades, or performance at work. Hypnosis can help mentally, for instance improving memory and increasing one's ability to concentrate. There is also evidence that hypnosis can help with pain relief and it has also been linked to helping break addictions such as smoking, alcoholism, and dependency on illegal drugs.

There's Absolutely Nothing To Worry About

On the whole, hypnosis is very safe, particularly when undertaken by a professional. Before visiting a hypnotherapist, it is advisable to research the individual or organization in question. Reports of hypnosis sessions going wrong are the responsibility of the hypnotherapist, and not the science itself. Sham hypnotists and poorly trained professionals can give a bad reputation to otherwise perfectly safe practice. Bear in mind, the hypnotist will have control of your mind, and therefore one should take due diligence when giving anyone that kind of responsibility.

Self Hypnosis Reveals More About Yourself

When dealing with your subconscious it is indeed very likely that repressed feelings and hidden motivations can surface. Very often we hide our true feelings about uncomfortable subjects, and when in a state of complete relaxation it is easier to connect with awkward emotions.

Hypnosis Can Alter One's Nature In The Long Term

Through regular practice, one can become more open to hypnotic suggestions, allowing for greater progress in one's chosen area of improvement. After a while of performing hypnosis, either self-induced or with a professional, one will be able to enter trance quicker and be more open to hypnotic suggestion. But never fear, this will not be the case for the rest of your life, and you will not become more easily influenced by just anybody. In fact, the more you are aware of how suggestions work, the better you will be at resisting other people's attempts at manipulating you.

Hypnosis Can Improve Sports Performance But Does Not Make You Physically Stronger

Although many people in sports use hypnosis to improve their game, let's be honest, hypnosis will not make you physically stronger. To gain the most from hypnosis, it is vital to understand what it can and can't do. When you have realistic expectations of hypnosis therapy you will gain greater benefits, for hoping for the impossible will only ever lead to disappointment. The change in performance relative to the sport may be bought on by one's increased confidence and fearless attitude. When one eliminates fear from one's life one can perform greater feats due to the release of mental limitations that were previously holding you back.

Is Hypnosis Real?

Hypnosis is a genuine psychological therapy process. It's often misunderstood and not widely used. However, medical research continues to clarify how and when hypnosis can be used as a therapy tool.

Fact Vs. Fiction: Busting 6 Popular Myths

Although hypnosis is slowly becoming more accepted in traditional medical practices, many myths about hypnosis persist. Here, we separate reality from falsehoods.

Myth: Everyone Can Be Hypnotized

Not everyone can be hypnotized. One study suggests that about 10 percent of the population is highly hypnotizable. Although it's possible that the rest of the population could be hypnotized, they're less likely to be receptive to the practice.

Myth: People Aren't In Control Of Their Body When They're Hypnotized

You're absolutely in control of your body during hypnosis. Despite what you see with stage hypnosis, you'll remain aware of what you're doing and what's being asked of you. If you don't want to do something you're asked to do under hypnosis, you won't do it.

Myth: Hypnosis Is The Same Thing As Sleep

You may look like you're sleeping, but you're awake during hypnosis. You're just in a deeply relaxed state. Your muscles will become limp, your breathing rate will slow, and you may become drowsy.

Myth: People Can't Lie When They're Hypnotized

Hypnotism isn't a truth serum. Although you're more open to suggestion during hypnotism, you still have free will and moral judgment. No one can make you say anything — lie or not — that you don't want to say.

Myth: You Can Be Hypnotized Over The Internet

Many smartphone apps and Internet videos promote self-hypnosis, but they're likely ineffective.

Probably A Myth: Hypnosis Can Help You "Uncover" Lost Memories

Although it may be possible to retrieve memories during hypnosis, you may be more likely to create false memories while in a trance-like state. Because of this, many hypnotists remain skeptical about using hypnosis for memory retrieval.

CHAPTER 2 - HYPNOSIS WEIGHT LOSS SESSION

Is One Session Enough?

Although one session can be helpful for some people, most therapists will tell you to begin hypnosis therapy with four to five sessions. After that phase, you can discuss how many more sessions are needed. You can also talk about whether any maintenance sessions are needed as well.

Hypnosis For Weight Loss

What is the link between hypnosis and weight loss? Hypnosis is something we typically think of as a type of entertainment but have you ever considered hypnosis for weight loss? It's easy to be skeptical of trying to use hypnosis to deal with a problem as serious as obesity, but maybe it's not as ridiculous as it sounds. Hypnosis for weight loss is certainly an appealing idea - it gives people a relatively easy out of their weight problem, by stopping their cravings for food at the source.

One problem with weight loss through hypnosis is the same problem that plagues other weight loss solutions. There are a lot of scams out there, and the people behind them will not think twice about trying to take your money for a product that doesn't do anything at all. Hypnosis has the same problem. You may be able to trust some claims about hypnosis weight loss therapy, but there are just as many ones that are full of lies.

The adage usually proves true in these situations: if something looks too good to be true, then it probably is. If hypnosis for weight loss treatment claims it can help you lose some crazy number of pounds in a couple of weeks or similar exaggerations, it's pretty safe to bet that it's a scam. If you find claims that state that hypnosis can completely alter the way the mind works to prevent eating, they're probably bogus.

However, the fact remains that hypnosis can help you lose weight. It's just that it won't cause those love handles to magically melt away overnight. Hypnosis is more science than magic - all it is when a person enters a state of deep, relaxed concentration in which they are more suggestible. This means that ideas put into a person's mind during a hypnosis session are much more likely to stick.

A session of hypnosis won't make you into some sort of robot that's immune to cravings and programmed not to overeat. What it can do, though, is make a person more likely to adhere to a proper dietary plan. The effects are entirely mental. Hypnosis can't "convince" your body to speed up weight loss, it can only implant the idea in your brain that maybe you don't need to eat that second piece of cake.

People seeking hypnotic solutions to weight loss should be especially careful of group hypnosis sessions. To work, hypnosis must be tailored specifically to the person receiving it. Group sessions clearly won't work, as the hypnotist cannot interact with any single person on his or her own. You should also be warned against hypnosis cassettes or videos, as they share this same issue.

Hypnosis for weight loss is a very tempting thought. If you can train your mind to reduce your cravings and increase your willpower, you'll be well on your way to losing weight. The important thing to remember is to be careful and study all the options before you buy a product or see a hypnotist, or else you might end with nothing at all.

Is Weight-Loss Hypnosis Effective?

Weight-loss hypnosis may help you shed an extra few pounds when it's part of a weight-loss plan that includes diet, exercise, and counseling. But it's hard to say definitively because there isn't enough solid scientific evidence about weight-loss hypnosis alone.

Hypnosis is a state of inner absorption and concentration, like being in a trance. Hypnosis is usually done with the help of a hypnotherapist using verbal repetition and mental images. When you're under hypnosis, your attention is highly focused, and you're more responsive to suggestions, including behavior changes that can help you lose weight.

A few studies have evaluated the use of weight-loss hypnosis. Most studies showed only slight weight loss, with an average loss of about 6 pounds (2.7 kilograms) over 18 months. But the quality of some of these studies has been questioned, making it hard to determine the true effectiveness of weight-loss hypnosis. However, a recent study, which only showed modest weight loss results, did find that patients receiving hypnosis had lower rates of inflammation, better satiety and better quality of life. These might be mechanisms whereby hypnosis could influence weight. Further studies are needed to fully understand the potential role of hypnosis in weight management. Weight loss is usually best achieved with diet and exercise. If you've tried diet and exercise but are still struggling to meet your weight-loss goal, talk to your health care provider about other options or lifestyle changes that you can make. Relying on weight-loss hypnosis alone is unlikely to lead to significant weight loss, but using it as an adjunct to an overall lifestyle approach may be worth exploring for some people.

Seeing Is Believing.

So see for yourself. You don't have to be entranced to learn some of the invaluable lessons that hypnosis has to teach about weight loss. The ten mini-concepts that follow contain some of the diet-altering suggestions my weight management clients receive in group and individual hypnotherapy.

1. **The Answer Lies Within:** Hypnotherapists believe you have everything you need to succeed. You don't need another crash diet or the latest appetite suppressant. Slimming is about trusting your innate abilities, as you do when you ride a bicycle. You may not remember how scary it was the first time you tried to bike, but you kept practicing until you could ride automatically, without thought or effort. Losing weight may seem similarly beyond you, but it's just a matter of finding your balance.

2. **Believing Is Seeing:** People tend to achieve what they think they can achieve. That even applies to hypnosis. Subjects tricked into believing they could be hypnotized (for example, as the hypnotist suggested they'd see red, he flipped the switch on a hidden red bulb) demonstrated increased hypnotic responsiveness. The expectation of being helped is essential. Let me suggest that you expect your weight loss plan to work.

3. **Accentuate The Positive:** Negative, or aversive, suggestions, like "Doughnuts will sicken you," work for a while, but if you want lasting change, you'll want to think positively. The most popular positive hypnotic suggestion was devised by doctors Herbert Spiegel and David Spiegel, a

father-son hypnotherapy team: "For my body, too much food is damaging. I need my body to live in. I owe my body respect and protection." I encourage clients to write their upbeat mantras. One 50-year-old mother who lost 50-plus pounds repeats daily: "Unnecessary food is a burden on my body. I'm going to shed what I don't need."

4. If You Imagine It, It Will Come: Like athletes preparing for competition, visualizing victory readies you for a victorious reality. Imagining a day of healthy eating helps you envision the necessary steps to becoming that healthy eater. Too tough to picture? Find an old photograph of yourself at a comfortable weight and remember what you were doing differently then; imagine resurrecting those routines. Or visualize getting advice from a future older, wiser self after she's reached her desired weight.

5. Send Food Cravings Flying: Hypnotherapists routinely harness the power of symbolic imagery, inviting subjects to put food cravings on fluffy white clouds or in hot air balloons and send them up, up, and away. If McDonald's golden arches have the power to steer you off your diet, hypnotists understand that a counter symbol can steer you back. Invite your mind to flip through its Rolodex of images until one emerges as a symbol for casting out cravings. Heave-ho.

6. Two Strategies Are Better Than One: When it comes to losing weight and keeping it off, a winning combination is a hypnosis and cognitive-behavioral therapy (CBT), which helps revamp counterproductive thoughts and behaviors. Clients who learn both lose twice as much weight without falling into the dieter's lose-some, regain-more trap. You've already tried CBT if you've ever kept a food diary. Before my clients learn hypnosis, they keep track of everything that passes their lips for a week or two. Raising awareness, every good hypnotherapist knows, is a key baby step toward lasting change.

7. Modify, Modify, Modify: The late hypnosis innovator Milton Erickson, MD, emphasized the importance of using existing patterns. To alter one client's lose-regain, lose-regain pattern, Erickson suggested she first gain weight before losing it—a hard sell nowadays, unless you're Charlize Theron. Easier to swallow: Modify your highest- calorie craving. Instead of a pint of ice cream, how about a cup of frozen yogurt?

8. Like It Or Not, It's Survival Of The Fattest: No suggestion is powerful enough to override the survival instinct. Much as we like to think it's survival of the fittest, we're still programmed, in case of famine, for the survival of the fattest. Case in point: a personal trainer on a starvation diet who wanted me to suggest a way her gummy bear addiction. I tried to explain that her body believed her life depended on the chewy candies and wouldn't give them up until she got enough calories from more nutritious foods. No, she insisted, a suggestion was all she needed. I wasn't surprised when she dropped out.

9. Practice Makes Perfect: One Pilates class does not produce washboard abs, and one hypnosis session cannot shape up your diet. But silently repeating a positive suggestion 15 to 20 minutes daily can transform your eating, especially when combined with slow, natural breaths, the cornerstone of any behavioral-change program.

10. Congrats It's A Relapse: When clients find themselves, against their healthiest intentions, overindulging, I congratulate them. Hypnosis views a relapse as an opportunity, not a travesty. If you can learn from a real or imagined relapse— why it happened, how to handle it differently—you'll be better prepared for life's inevitable temptations.

How To Use Hypnosis To Change Eating Habits

Let Hypnosis Control Your Eating Habits To Lose Weight, Even Permanently

Controlling your eating habits is tasking and difficult. But, if your body needs to be trimmed down because of being overweight, you don't have the choice, but to cut appetite, reduce the volume of food you eat. If we look into some of the common ways of diet programs, there are many which are practically applicable, and may even be effective if we are just diligent in doing its process.

The need for proper control of your diet is essential to losing weight. But this entails a lot of effort to do and maintain since you need to endure from abstaining to eat what you wanted to eat. Taking the diet program is directly against your eating habits. It is the primary reason why diet programs won't last long, and the need to lose weight would eventually fail. If you were able to maintain the habit of abstaining to eat too much, could you endure in subjecting yourself to the process? How long?

Diet program, if only maintained, is already beneficial. You can already eliminate fats, and trim down into a good body shape. But you must exert effort and hold on to sustain from denying yourself the adverse attitudes and the bad eating habits that you are used to. But, with hypnosis, to lose weight by controlling the eating habit, bad eating habits, will just go easy and will be far off different from what we could imagine from our discussions above. All of these losing weight programs will be turning to a smoothly easy method of exercise and diet programs, and you will eventually be used to it the easy way.

Study shows that in hypnosis you are not brought directly to the actual abstinence from your bad eating habits, or follow strictly the diet programs. Hypnosis is a method that goes first to the mental faculties of a person. Hypnosis entails conditioning of the mind which will eventually develop a behavioral attitude and transform the physical condition and habits that we are used to, depending upon the series of preliminary instructions and suggestions induced to the mind for whatever physical condition or habit or behavior it is intended for. With the hypnotic method of weight loss program, such as that of the above, a person's behavior is already set in the mind, and the physical attributes and the used to habits are changed and reformed to regularly practice and maintain weight lose program, the exercise, and diets, naturally, done as easy as the natural course of the lifestyle of the person.

Losing weight by controlling eating habits with hypnosis is much more effective, being a natural, formed and practiced as used to daily habits, with the long-lasting permanent result, good health and a body shaped up, trimmed and attractive

Using Hypnosis In Different Ways

Hypnosis is a state where the mind thinks and directs the body to play an imaginative role. As opposed to popular belief, hypnosis is not a condition of unconsciousness. The body is put in a relaxed state by intensified mental concentration induced by another person or even self-administered. Hypnosis is accepted and practiced by experts.

Nonetheless, inexperienced hypnotists are cautioned for possible backfires. It doesn't work all the time even for specialists. Not all people can be hypnotists and as it follows, not all can be easily hypnotized.

Inducing hypnosis can help you see through a person's mind. During daily conversations, you can have someone reveal to you his deepest secrets without him realizing it. Furthermore, you can change his opinions and direct how he responds to questions. There is a set of words, known as the 'hot words', used to better hypnotize people. Studying these words will help, most especially when trying to influence more than one person. Aside from the 'hot words', making a hypnotic story is also a good move. These techniques are easy to master with due practice.

But what do we get from learning to hypnotize? You can evade a big debt and even solicit money from the person you owe or get a prospective investor to sign a bogus contract. Hypnosis can give you money, yes, but contrary to what the majority believes, hypnotizing is not only about profiteering.

It can be used as self-defense. During dangerous situations, more so if you don't have any knowledge of martial arts, you can use hypnosis on your perpetrator. Putting yourself in a trance is also a good form of resting. It can give you the peace you seek even in the noisiest places. Hypnosis also aids in the development of the brain. If you have mastered this art, your mind gains faster reactions even to daily activities such as analyzing the content of a very technical text. For instructors, sometimes it is easy to teach a lesson, but the students just lack the right motivation. You can provide them the needed drive through hypnosis.

Most of all, knowing how to instigate hypnotism, will eventually help you counter hypnosis when induced on you. Have you ever walked down an alley and then found yourself giving a huge sum of money to someone you don't even know? Or perhaps getting out of your car and giving some stranger your key? This means you can be a vulnerable target; thus, you also need to learn how to hypnotize. Hypnosis is more accurately defined as the ability to preeminent others' will power. It can be either harmful or beneficial depending on how you use and how you conduct it.

Hypnosis Is The Key To Your Mind And Your Health!

Our mind is the center of a very complex nervous system. Networks of nerve cells run throughout the body, connecting every tissue to our brain. Electrical impulses travel along these pathways at high speeds, leaping across narrow gaps between cells, relaying information to and from our mind. Our mind itself has two parts, a conscious and subconscious. Most of us are pretty familiar with the conscious mind. It organizes and runs our outer life. But many of our decisions that affect our life come from our subconscious. The subconscious is very powerful and has many functions.

1. Serves As A Memory Bank: Here in the brain with the help of billions of tiny interconnected nerve cells, everything that we have ever experienced is stored. The subconscious is the very cells of the body storing a maze of memory patterns which, when activated will feed information to the conscious mind. Nothing is ever erased unless the computer in the subconscious mind gives that command.

2. Controls And Regulates The Involuntary Functions Of The Body: These are breathing, circulation, metabolism, digestion, hormone balance, etc. Hypnosis is used to affect these areas.

3. The Subconscious In The Seat Of Our Emotions: Since our emotions govern the strength of our desires, and these affect our behavior, many behavior issues have very strong emotional content. Hypnosis is used to release stored emotions.

4. It Is The Home Of The Imagination: Even when we're not using it, each of us has a strong and active imagination that can be used in a positive way to create our goals. Creative visualization done in trance is one of the greatest secrets of success.

5. It Carries Out Habitual Conduct: Through the use of direct & indirect suggestions in hypnosis, we can create a system of habits that support and create our goals.

6. The Subconscious Is The Dynamo That Directs Our Energy, And Drives Us Towards Our Goals: It generates and releases energy, and if it's not consciously directed, it is directed by circumstances and chance. Through positive reprogramming, the subconscious is directed towards creating our goals. Hypnosis is the most practical and effective way to enter the subconscious mind, which is very suggestible when you talk to it in the right way. Hypnotherapists are people who are trained to work with hypnosis to help people create positive changes in their lives. The field of hypnotherapy stretches from traditional work with weight, smoking and stress to clinical (medical) use of hypnosis. In the clinical field, hypnosis has been very effective in working with head injuries, pain management, and life-threatening diseases.

Self Hypnosis is a wonderful way to start creating positive changes in your life. The best way to learn is actually in trance. Go into trance using the following formula: "Close your eyes, take in three deep breaths, count backward from ten to one, relax your body, relax your mind... you will be in a deep state of hypnosis." anchor "every time you want to practice your self-hypnosis close your eyes, take in three deep breaths, count backward from ten to one, relax your mind and you will be in a deep state of hypnosis." Begin your suggestions and your visualization.

Guidelines For Suggestions:

1. Motivation and desire must be strong before you use a suggestion to think about why you want it to happen.

2. Always be positive and enthusiastic.

3. Always use the present tense, imagine yourself achieving the goal now.

4. Suggest action; see yourself in the act of doing what you want.

5. Be specific.

6. Keep the language simple and direct.

7. Fuel visualizations and suggestions with positive emotions.

8. Use repetition especially of keywords and phrases.

9. Bring yourself back to waking consciousness.

You can easily learn this, and once you master this technique, you open the door to great potential. It has been estimated that the average human being uses 3 to 7% of their mind's capacity. By using hypnosis you can learn to operate your wonderful bio-computer. Your mind holds the key to your health.

CHAPTER 3 - A BASIC SELF-HYPNOSIS SESSION FOR WEIGHT LOSS

Self-Hypnosis: What It Is And What It Can Do

Hypnosis is the practice of promoting an altered state of mind or consciousness where patients become highly responsive to suggestions by the person performing the hypnosis. It is often used in psychiatric and medical treatments. Hypnosis is characterized by repetitive vocal suggestions and commands that are uttered in a monotonous tone of voice. The sound is meant to induce relaxation and calmness by focusing on the patient's consciousness on a specific subject or idea.

With the use of self-hypnosis to achieve a better life, the act is performed by the patient himself, usually through the aid of a picture, video or audio recording. Sometimes, self-hypnosis that is similar to meditation may also be used. This is accompanied by controlled breathing exercises and repetitive verbal self commands.

Why Self-Hypnosis?

There are a variety of reasons why people turn to self-hypnosis to achieve a better life. Often, it is used as an alternative therapy to supplement other treatments such as psychotherapy or medication and may also be used in conjunction with medical issues. People often turn to self-hypnosis because they prefer the privacy it affords. Self-hypnosis also allows them to be more flexible with their time. Aside from that, self-hypnosis usually turns out to be a less costly investment, since there are no expensive hypno-therapist fees to pay for.

What Types Of Techniques Are Often Used In Self-Hypnosis For A Better Life?

Aided self-hypnosis is probably the most common technique, using tools such as visual aids, tapes, and videos, although much-advanced users may prefer self-command. Most self-hypnosis experts agree that people who practice self-hypnosis for a better life are better off using beginner or basic techniques. Advanced techniques are often more difficult and complicated and will require the guidance of a trained professional.

How Is It Supposed To Work?

Self-hypnosis for a better life uses positive suggestions to appeal to the unconscious mind, promoting feelings of self-worth and well being. By keeping the body and mind relaxed and reducing stress, distractions are eliminated and positive suggestions are focused on. When these suggestions are magnified, the self-hypnotism begins to accept it as the truth, applying it to his life after the self-hypnosis session is over.

Does It Always Work?

Self-hypnosis to achieve a better life is a form of self-help that is resorted to willingly by people who wish to experience an improvement in their lives. It is wise to note, however, that not all people can be hypnotized because not all of us are prone to believing or accepting suggestions. As for helping people achieve a better life, self-hypnosis has had mixed results. People who have tried to sustain self-hypnosis sessions and attain a hypnotic state of mind have reported feelings of calmness, relaxation, peace and well being. These emotions often pave the way for the development of self-esteem. With self-esteem, most people become more willing to open themselves to changing their lives, accepting and implementing improvements.

On the other hand, most people who use self-hypnosis without success are often those who are incapable of sustaining the practice, participating in the sessions intermittently. Also, people who have difficulty concentrating or keeping their focus usually report no improvement.

Hypnosis And Self Hypnosis For Weight Loss

The notion of using hypnosis or self-hypnosis for weight loss is certainly intriguing, and one that would be nice to believe in, but is it for real? The idea isn't quite as farfetched as it used to be since today more people are familiar with how the subconscious mind works. Hypnosis and self-hypnosis are now used for a variety of purposes, and while not yet exactly mainstream, the idea is at least accepted as possible by many. Strictly speaking, no one is saying that you can't make pounds disappear by hypnosis, as though by magic. No, hypnosis is designed to reprogram your subconscious mind so that you behave differently. After all, your actions have a lot to do with your weight, as well as many other aspects of your physical health. Put like that, it doesn't seem so hard to believe.

So What Kind Of Changes Can Hypnosis Cause In Our Behavior?

- ❖ Eat Less: Consume fewer calories
- ❖ Eat Healthier: Make better choices when shopping/ordering out
- ❖ Exercise More: More motivation when exercising
- ❖ Improved Self Image: Reduce self-sabotage

Can hypnosis do all these things? Theoretically, yes. Does it always work this well for everyone who tries it?

Unfortunately, no. But, then, nothing works for everybody, including diets, exercise or diet pills.

What Is Hypnosis Anyway?

"Hypnosis" is a relatively new word, having been coined in the 19th Century based on the work of a man named Franz Mesmer (from whom we got the word "mesmerism" which means the same thing as hypnosis). It means going into a trance state where you are highly suggestible. In more recent times, scientists have identified certain specific brain waves that occur during such states.

Hypnosis was originally associated with stage hypnotists and magicians, who would make people do funny or bizarre things under hypnosis. Yet at the same time, it was also being used for therapeutic purposes. It fit in well with the emerging field of psychology, which emphasized the role of the subconscious mind in our behavior.

Using Hypnosis For Weight Loss

If you wanted to lose weight using hypnosis, how would you go about it? Well, you could visit a qualified hypnotherapist. While this wouldn't be cheap, compared to any type of traditional therapy, it has the advantage of being fast-acting. Most hypnotherapists focus on teaching you techniques you can use on your own, so you don't have to constantly return to them for sessions.

Another option is to find one of the many recordings that are designed to help you lose weight. These can be played at your convenience, though you can't play them while driving or doing anything where your full conscious attention is required.

One Tool Among Many

Don't expect hypnosis to work all by itself. Of course, the whole point is that it's supposed to make it easier for you to stick to your diet, exercise program, and other goals. However, your conscious mind has to help it along by trying your best to stay focused.

Since hypnosis focuses on your subconscious, it's still up to you to find the external tools that work best for you. In other words, you should do your research and find a healthy diet and that agrees with your body (not all diets work well for every person).

The same is true for exercise. If you've always hated going to the gym, you shouldn't try to hypnotize yourself into loving it. Work with your natural tendencies, and get yourself to exercise in a way that's consistent with your interests and preferences.

The real objective of hypnosis for weight loss is to allow you to do the things that you have to do to lose weight without having to exert so much will power. If your subconscious mind is more in alignment with your conscious goals, there's less of a chance that you'll sabotage yourself by cheating on your diet or abandoning your exercise program.

Using hypnosis to lose weight may sound strange or exotic, but it's just another way to use your mind in a way that supports your goals. It may not be for everyone, but if the idea sounds appealing or at least interesting, you may want to look into some of the possibilities for losing weight using hypnosis.

How To Self-Hypnotize For Weight Loss

The process of hypnosis is getting your mind into a state where it can accept a suggestion. During hypnosis, a subject can take a trip deep into their subconscious to eliminate beliefs and habits that may be a detriment to his everyday life. This is why hypnosis is so popular for those seeking to lose weight. However, it is not necessary to seek and pay for a professional. Most insurance plans also do not cover the cost of hypnotherapy. Try to self-hypnotize yourself to lose extra weight.

Step 1

Find Time In Your Day Where You Will Not Be Distracted By External Factors: Try to set aside at least 30 minutes where you can immerse yourself in a trance. It is important to focus during this entire period.

Step 2

Set Weight Loss Goals For Yourself: Aim for an exact amount of weight you want to lose and a specific time you want to lose it. Read this goal aloud before you begin.

Step 3

Visualize Yourself As The Size You Want To Be: Imagine what your body will look like once you attain your ideal weight. Also, think about how others will react and what they will say. Try to make the scene as vivid as possible rich with color, smells, sounds, and feelings.

Step 4

Close Your Eyes And Relax Your Body Until It Is Completely Limp: Engage in deep breathing for three minutes until you feel a sensation from your skull to your feet. After the sensation is felt, relax that part of your body. You will be in a trance state.

Step 5

Imagine Your Ideal Self In A Trance State: Think about how you will view the world, the way others will see you, and how good it will feel to be healthy and in good shape. Look at your body in its lean, trim state.

Step 6

Come Back To Your Present State Slowly: Be sure you bring the feelings of the internal experience back with you. Doing this daily will train your mind to feel how good it will be to lose weight. You will gradually make the behavior modifications necessary to lose weight.

As you may see, I have put together a Complete Weight Loss Program for you based on feedback from my Weight Loss Classes. This course is specially designed to Empower You on your successful Weight Loss journey. Please ensure that you do not listen to the Hypnosis sessions whilst driving or working.

The Thirteen Hypnosis Sessions Are :

1. **Boost Your Metabolism:** You will take a journey into a beautiful garden, whereby you will visit your unconscious mind control panel and Increase The Speed Of Your Metabolism.

2. **Create An Image Of The Ideal You:** In this Hypnosis session, you will visit a wonderful lake and see your reflection change into the person you will become. This image will stay with you and Become Your Goal.

3. **Eliminate Your Bad Eating Habits:** You will visit a lovely beach, there you will find a treasure chest and you will place within it a symbol representing each of

your bad eating habits, then Bury The Chest, And Your Bad Eating Habits.

4. **Receiving The Hypnotic Gastric Band:** This is a great session, you will visit a clinic and meet a lovely nurse who will look after you throughout. You will experience the procedure as an observer looking down on yourself, No Discomfort and No Anxiety.

5. **Adjusting The Hypnotic Gastric Band:** In this session, you will revisit the clinic and have the Hypnotic Gastric Band adjusted so that you will feel full whilst eating less, another great hypnosis session.

6. **Motivation To Exercise:** This Hypnosis session will assist you to exercise, even if it is only walking. As you know the hardest part of anything, is getting started.

7. **Self Esteem & Confidence:** Not only do you want to look good, but you also need to feel great. This hypnosis session will help you do just that.

8. **Emotional Eating:** How many times have you reached for something to eat when you are feeling down. This session will help to stop you from Comfort Eating.

9. **Healthy Eating:** To ensure your continuing weight loss, and to keep it going, you must ensure a healthy eating

lifestyle. This session will assist you in Stopping Eating Fatty Foods.
10. **Maintaining Your Weight Loss:** After putting in all the hard work, the last thing you want to do is put it back on again. This Hypnosis session will help you stay on track.
11. **Chocolate Addiction:** This first Bonus Session will assist in the battle against Eating Too Much Chocolate.
12. **Sugar Addiction:** This second Bonus Session will assist you in Controlling Your Sugar Intake.
13. **Alcohol-Related Weight Gain:** This session will assist you in Lowering Your Alcohol Intake.

Next Session To Be Added "Stop Night Time Snacking"

Each Hypnosis session begins with a beautiful hypnotic total body relaxation, allowing you to drift into a wonderful deep relaxed state.

Self Hypnosis For Weight Loss- 7 Huge Benefits For You

Self-hypnosis for weight loss is a fantastic self-help tool that can help you shed those extra few pounds and change your life for the better if you have been struggling with losing weight for a while. In this article, I will give you a summary of the seven biggest benefits weight loss through self-hypnosis can bring you.

Self-Hypnosis For Weight Loss

1. You Can Practice Self Hypnosis For Weight Loss From The Comfort Of Your Own Home: People prefer doing self-hypnosis at home for a variety of reasons:

- ❖ Some people are just too busy between work and family commitments to fit in appointments.
- ❖ Some people don't have access to transport.
- ❖ Some people who are overweight find it hard to get around.
- ❖ Sometimes people with excess weight can feel ashamed of their bodies and don't want to be seen.

If any of these reasons apply to you, working towards weight loss at home might suit you down to the ground.

2. Save Your Hard Earned Money

Two arguments for using hypnotic weight loss:

- ❖ Weight loss hypnosis compares favorably in terms of outcomes to run-of-the-mill weight loss programs.
- ❖ Weight loss through hypnosis is backed by scientific research.

One potential downside:

Hypnosis comes at a higher cost than most conventional weight loss programs. This higher cost can be an obstacle to people accessing hypnotherapy.

Using self-hypnosis for weight loss will enable you to do the suggestion hypnosis part of your weight loss program for very little money. If you wanted to, you could even design your self-hypnosis program and do the whole lot for free.

When you compare this to the commitment of seeing a weight loss hypnotist for maybe eight appointments over the space of a year, self-hypnosis for weight loss represents a substantial saving.

If you are an emotional eater or are planning to lose a substantial amount of weight, I would still recommend you back up the suggestion program with some regression hypnosis to remove the underlying causes of weight issues.

3. Self Hypnosis For Weight Loss Is Both Easy And Effective

Self-hypnosis is easy to learn, enjoyable to practice and very effective. What could be more enjoyable than breaking your busy lifestyle with periods of relaxation where you can lie back and let go while working towards weight loss?

With self-hypnosis, there is no 'efforting' and no struggle. The underlying principle is about convincing your subconscious mind to come on board with your weight loss plan. This means generating determination and an abundance of positive feelings towards the idea of losing weight. This approach can put people miles ahead of those who struggle in conventional weight loss programs. Self-hypnosis for weight loss can take the struggle out of weight loss when complex decisions become easy because your mind is set on your goal.

4. Be Independent With Self Hypnosis For Weight Loss

Self-hypnosis allows you to be independent. No appointments, no practitioner. Just you. With self-hypnosis, you will act as both hypnotist and client. This feature will be particularly important for you if you don't like the idea of handing over your mind to a weight loss hypnotist. Self-help hypnosis can have some challenges, but there are ways of mastering those and achieving the same or similar results you can achieve by working with a hypnotist.

There is a saying that goes: **"Self Help is the Best Form of Help".**

I think this takes on a special meaning for self-hypnosis. My observation is that when people take charge to do things for themselves, they are more invested in both process and outcome. As a result, when using self-hypnosis to lose weight, you will notice yourself becoming very determined and motivated to see this process until you reach your goal.

5. You Can Use Self Hypnosis Whenever It Suits You

A self-hypnosis program can fit into your busy lifestyle easily. Some exercises can be done when multitasking, for example when you are doing a monotonous task such as washing the dishes, while you are walking, or commuting to work. Another exercise will require a little bit of space where you are undisturbed, but 20 minutes a day will already bring you a long way here. If- as part of your self-hypnosis program, you are planning to listen to a recorded hypnotherapy session, you can do this at bedtime while you are settling. Scheduling the hypnosis session in this way can help you work around your parenting responsibilities if you have kids.

6. Be In Complete Control

If you don't like the idea of handing over your mind to a hypnotherapist, working with self-hypnosis for weight loss may be just the thing for you. With self-hypnosis, you avoiding the issue of making yourself dependent on a practitioner. Here, you can be in complete control of your weight loss program. Among other things, self-hypnosis will give you control over:

- ❖ The content of your self-hypnosis program
- ❖ Which exercises you use- choose those you like best
- ❖ Where and when you practice

❖ Being in complete control will enable you to make every aspect of your program suit your personal needs and wants.

7. Gain Self Help Tools For Life

When you use self-hypnosis for weight loss you will learn a variety of tools. You will develop a good sense of which ones you like better than others. You will choose those you prefer and you will learn to make them work for you. Once you have reached your weight loss goal, you can apply these tools to any other changes you might want to make in your life. Learning self-hypnosis is a skill for life. I use self-hypnosis myself daily. It helps me master various challenges and wouldn't want to be without it.

CHAPTER 4 - HYPNOSIS PORTION CONTROL SESSION

Control And Start Eating The Right Amount

Portion control can play a significant role in achieving your health and weight goals. You may already be eating all the right foods and taking appropriate exercise. But if you still find yourself carrying excess weight, it could be because you are simply consuming too much. Portion control can make a big difference. Good portion control won't just make you slimmer - it gives you more energy. Eating the right amount will mean your body has to work less hard to digest unnecessary excess food.

Portion Control Is About The Right Amount Of Food

Quantity is as important as quality when it comes to getting your diet right and shedding excess fat. Too much of a good thing really can be bad for you when you need to lose weight. Yet it can feel hard to knowhow, when, and how much to cut down so that you can begin to see some progress in reaching your weight goals.

Why Is It So Hard To Exercise Portion Control?

Habit rules our lives much more than we realize. We eat because it's time to eat (even though you had a snack just half an hour ago). We overeat out of politeness, or not wanting to 'waste' what is on our plate, or just because we are so used to stuffing ourselves that we have forgotten how to recognize when we've had enough. Of course, some common sense things can help you control portion size:

- ❖ You can consciously eat more slowly: This gives your stomach a chance to register its fullness in your brain and switch off your appetite.
- ❖ You can start your meal with soup - A low-calorie soup can be very satisfying and allow you to feel happy with a much smaller portion of your main course.
- ❖ You can use the old smaller plate trick: So you have to eat smaller portions.
- ❖ You can avoid buffets and ignore 'mega-meal' deals.

Hypnosis Is A Powerful Tool For Portion Control

But great as all of the above advice is, you still need to overcome habit and compulsion - and that's where hypnosis can help. Food is fuel, and fuel needs to be of the right quality and quantity. Imagine trying to put more fuel into your car when it's already full. It just doesn't make sense.

Portion control will take you into a deeply relaxed state and quickly train your unconscious mind to know instinctively when to leave excess food alone and allow your digestion to be so much more comfortable. You will rediscover the pleasure of being in tune with what your own body needs for nourishment.

Why Is Portion Control Difficult?

Our habits rule our lives we eat for many more reasons than we are required to. We eat:

- Because high sugar and sodium "invite" us to do so, satisfying our need for more
- Because we are used to stuffing ourselves
- Out of politeness
- Not wanting to waste
- Because we've forgotten how much is enough
- Because we are bored, depressed, or angry

Portion Control Plays A Significant Role In Your Life

You already may be eating all the right foods and exercising, but if you still find yourself carrying extra weight or pounds that just won't shed, it could be that you are simply consuming too much. Portion control makes all the difference.

Correct Portion Control Affects Your Energy And Metabolism

Controlling your portions when eating doesn't just make you slimmer, it is also a trigger mechanism in your body that gives you more energy and increases your metabolism. When the body has too much food "thrown at it" your body has to work hard to digest and absorb unnecessary food. This takes extra energy and causes your metabolism to slow down as your body puts up a defensive mechanism.

Overcome Habit And Compulsion Issues With Hypnosis For Portion Control

You need to overcome the habit and compulsion involved in portion control issues and that's where hypnosis is an effective tool. Hypnosis for portion control takes you into a deeply relaxed mode and retrains your subconscious mind to instinctively leave excess food behind, allowing your metabolism to increase because a reasonable amount of food is being given to the body. Rediscover the enjoyment of being in tune with your body and without that uncomfortable, heavy feeling after you eat and "it happened again...I ate too much."

See how hypnosis can significantly impact the direction of your life. Become more and more focused on your goals, make progress, enjoy a greater feeling of self-worth and satisfaction and see more results from your progress — it's all possible with hypnosis.

Why Hypnosis Is A Powerful Tool For Portion Control

Great as all of the above advice is, you still need to overcome habit and compulsion - and that's where hypnosis can help.

Food is fuel, and fuel needs to be of the right quality and quantity. Imagine trying to put more fuel into your car when it's already full. It just doesn't make sense.

The Portion Control hypnosis session will take you into a deeply relaxed state and quickly train your unconscious mind to know instinctively when to leave excess food alone and allow your digestion to be so much more comfortable. You will rediscover the pleasure of being in tune with what your own body needs for nourishment.

What Is Overeating? How To Control Your Portions

Portion control is an essential component of a healthy lifestyle. But you might wonder how to put the idea into practice. What is overeating? How can you stop? To maintain a healthy diet, it's important to recognize signs you've eaten too much and learn to limit portion sizes

What Is Overeating?

Overeating refers to eating more calories than your body uses for energy. People sometimes overeat for emotional or psychological reasons, such as boredom, anxiety, depression, or stress.

To figure out whether you're eating too much, first review the correct amount of daily calories needed for your weight, age, metabolism, physical activity level, and gender. For instance, a 150-pound woman who works out regularly needs more calories than a woman of the same size who rarely exercises.

Overeating can lead to a host of health problems, including obesity, heart disease, high blood pressure, and high cholesterol. That's why it's important to get your food portions under control.

Signs You've Eaten Too Much

Ask yourself how you feel after eating. Are you uncomfortable and bloated? Stomach discomfort feeling gassy and/or swollen is a major sign of overeating. Also, if you overeat, you may feel embarrassed or distressed after finishing a meal. People who overeat may feel that they lack control over what and how much they consume. A history of failed diets could also indicate that you struggle with overeating. Frequent overeating may indicate binge eating disorder (BED). Common signs of BED include eating faster than normal, eating until you're uncomfortably full, eating alone often, or consuming large amounts of food when you're not hungry. If you regularly notice signs you've eaten too much, it may help to work with your doctor or dietitian to make a healthier meal plan.

How To Stop Overeating

Now that you've answered the "am I overeating?" question, it's time to take action. An initial step is keeping track of what you eat. Record your meals and snacks including when, why, and how much you eat to help control your food portions. Reading food labels to check calories per serving, along with creating a food tracker. This tracker can be kept on your phone, as part of an online calendar, or in a notebook. It will help you discover the details of your eating habits and note your progress.

These Tips For Managing Portions At Home:

- Eat one serving, according to the food label or recipe
- Eat your food slowly to let your brain get the message that your stomach is full
- Exchange large plates and glasses for smaller ones to help you eat and drink less
- Fill your plate with mostly low-calorie foods and foods low in saturated fat
- Eat your meals at the same times every day eating at different times or skipping meals may lead to overeating later in the day

Also watch your portions at restaurants, which tend to serve more food than you need. Share a meal with a friend, avoid buffets, skip the bread and chips, or simply choose healthier, lighter food options on the menu.

CHAPTER 5 - GASTRIC BAND HYPNOTHERAPY

Gastric band hypnotherapy is a technique used to suggest to the subconscious that you've had a gastric band fitted around your stomach, to help you lose weight. Considered a last resort, gastric band surgery involves fitting a band around the upper part of the stomach. This limits the amount of food you can physically eat, encouraging weight loss. It's a surgical procedure and therefore comes with potential risks and complications.

Gastric band hypnotherapy or having a 'virtual gastric band' fitted doesn't require surgery. It is a technique used by hypnotherapists to get the subconscious to believe there's been a gastric band fitted. The aim is that on an unconscious level, you will believe that you've had the physical procedure and that your stomach has reduced in size. The process doesn't involve surgery or medication and is completely safe. On this page, we will explore what gastric band hypnotherapy involves, how it works and whether or not it could work for you.

What Is A Gastric Band?

A gastric band is an adjustable silicone device used in weight loss surgery. The band is placed around the upper section of the stomach to create a small pouch above the device. This restricts the amount of food that can be stored in the stomach, making it difficult to eat large amounts. A gastric band aims to restrict the amount of food a person can physically eat, causing them to feel full after eating very little to encourage weight loss. For most people who have this surgery, it is the last resort after trying other methods of weight loss. Like any surgery, fitting a gastric band comes with risks.

Gastric Band Hypnosis

Gastric band hypnosis can be used to help people lose weight, without the risks that come with surgery. Many hypnotherapists use a two-pronged approach. First, they look to identify the root cause of your emotional eating.

Using hypnosis, the therapist can encourage you to remember long-forgotten experiences surrounding food that maybe subconsciously affecting you now. Addressing and recognizing any unhealthy thought patterns surrounding food can be helpful before carrying out gastric band hypnotherapy.

Next, the hypnotherapist will carry out the virtual gastric band treatment. The procedure is designed to suggest, at a subconscious level, that you have had an operation to insert a gastric band. The aim is for your body to respond to this suggestion by making you feel fuller quicker as if you had the real surgery.

Hypnotherapist Becca Teers Explains Why Diets Don't Work For Weight Loss:

"Diets don't tend to deal with the permanent lifestyle changes required, such as a sustainable long-term change in our eating habits and attitude to food. Many diet plans are temporary and can be difficult to maintain on an on-going basis, often because they are too restrictive or they deprive us of our favorite foods. These regimes can be adhered to short-term but don't work so well in the long run. By causing us to count calories or consciously measure portion size or even totally omit types of foods, many diets can make us more obsessed with food and our eating. This can take the pleasure out of eating and can lead us to crave more of certain foods and a diet-overeat/binge cycle can start."

The Benefits

A gastric band is considered to be the safest weight loss surgery. It's a relatively simple low risk minimally invasive procedure with few complications. Gastric band surgery usually results in a shorter hospital stay (just one night), a faster recovery time (approximately one week), smaller scars and less pain than other gastric surgery procedures.

Unlike with a gastric bypass and a sleeve gastrectomy, a gastric band involves no permanent alteration to your body such as removing part of your stomach or re-routing and stapling your body. It is completely reversible and can be removed if desired. Having a gastric band fitted doesn't interfere with the digestion and absorption of your food. Vitamin deficiencies and dumping syndrome often associated with gastric bypass surgery are less likely to occur with a gastric band and you shouldn't need to take daily nutritional supplements. Band adjustments can easily be done quickly in your surgeon's clinic or hospital as required to help you keep on track with your weight loss.

Gastric bands offer a more gradual weight loss than other gastric surgeries. Weighing less makes it much easier for you to move around and do your everyday activities as well as join in new activities that can help improve your general fitness and wellbeing. Weight loss with a gastric band will lead to improvements in co-morbid conditions related to obesity, including type 2 diabetes, high cholesterol, sleep apnoea, and high blood pressure.

After significant weight loss following a gastric banding procedure, you may feel an improvement in your psychological welfare, with the higher self- and body esteem, less depressive symptoms and a better quality of life.

What Are The Risks?

The insertion of a gastric band is a surgical procedure and, although rare, carries potential risks. There are also some gastric band side effects worth noting.

The main complications that can occur following gastric weight loss surgery include infection, blood clots in the legs (deep vein thrombosis) or lungs (pulmonary embolism) and internal bleeding.

Generally, one in ten people with a gastric band will need a further operation at some time in the future. This may be for several reasons. Your wound, port or band may become infected and may need to be re-sited, replaced or removed. Sometimes, very slowly, your band can work its way into or through the wall of your stomach so that it's ineffective and would need to be removed and replaced. There is a risk that over time your band slips out of position and your stomach pouch will become enlarged. Your gastric band would need re-fixing in the correct position. Components of your gastric band may come apart due to damage and cause it to leak. The damaged part would need to be replaced. Some people with a gastric band develop a food intolerance resulting in symptoms such as nausea, vomiting and gastro-oesophageal reflux (GER). In most cases, avoiding foods that trigger a reaction should help, but if you have persistent symptoms associated with several different foods, it may be necessary to remove the band. People who lose a lot of weight, regardless of the gastric weight loss surgery, are at high risk of developing gallstones.

How Gastric Band Hypnosis Works

Using relaxation techniques a hypnotherapist will put you into a state of hypnosis. In this relaxed state, your subconscious is more open to suggestion. At this point, hypnotherapists make suggestions to your subconscious. With gastric band hypnotherapy, this suggestion is that you've had a physical band fitted. The mind is powerful, so if you're subconscious accepts these suggestions, your behavior will change accordingly. Usually, along with the 'fitting' of the virtual gastric band, suggestions surrounding confidence and behavior will be made to help you commit to this change in lifestyle.

Many therapists will also teach self-hypnosis techniques so you can enhance the work you've done following the session. Educating yourself on nutrition and exercise is often advised as well, to promote physical health and well-being.

The Procedure

Your first meeting with the hypnotherapist will likely be an initial consultation where you discuss what you hope to gain from hypnotherapy. This is an opportunity to talk about any previous weight loss attempts, your eating habits, any health issues and your general attitude towards food. This information will give the therapist a clearer idea of what will help and whether or not any other forms of treatment should be considered. The procedure itself is designed to mimic gastric band surgery, to help your subconscious believe it has happened. To make the experience more authentic, many hypnotherapists will incorporate the sounds and smells of an operating theatre. Your therapist will begin by taking you into a deeply relaxed state, also known as hypnosis. You will be aware of what is happening and will be in control at all times.

Once you are in a hypnotic state, the therapist will talk you through the operation. They will explain step by step what happens in surgery, from being put under the anesthetic, to make the first incision, fitting the band itself and stitching up the cut. Sounds and smells of an operating theatre will enhance the experience, to persuade your subconscious that what's being said is happening to you. As previously mentioned, other suggestions may be incorporated during the procedure to increase self-confidence. Once the procedure is complete, your hypnotherapist may teach you some self-hypnosis techniques to help you stay on track at home.

Some hypnotherapists will request that you return for follow-up appointments to monitor the virtual band's success and to make any adjustments. This happens when people get the physical band fitted too. For some, it can be helpful to continue hypnotherapy sessions as part of a long-term weight management plan. This allows the hypnotherapist to work with you to address underlying issues surrounding food and self-esteem.

Gastric band hypnosis should form part of a weight management program that addresses nutrition and exercise habits. It is the combination of changing habits in both body and mind that is often most successful for those seeking weight loss.

How Will I Feel After?

The overall aim of gastric band hypnosis is to encourage a healthier relationship with food. When your subconscious believes you have had a gastric band fitted, it will believe your stomach is smaller. This, in turn, makes your brain send out messages that you are full after consuming less food. For those who overeat, recognizing when you're physically full can be difficult. Sometimes we eat purely for the taste (or comfort), ignoring whether or not we are physically hungry. Learning to recognize the physical sensations of being hungry and being full helps cultivate healthy eating habits. Unlike gastric band surgery, the virtual gastric band does not have any physical side-effects. For some, the real surgery can cause nausea, vomiting and acid reflux. As gastric band hypnosis isn't a physical process, it won't cause symptoms like this.

Will It Work For Me?

A common question for those trying hypnotherapy for the first time is - will it work for me? Unfortunately, it isn't a simple case of yes or no; it is largely up to you. Hypnotherapy helps people with a range of concerns but is particularly useful when it comes to changing habits. For this reason, it is often successful in helping people develop healthy eating habits and lose weight. However, just like any other weight loss system, it will require your total commitment.

You are more likely to get what you want from gastric band hypnotherapy if you believe in the process and your therapist. Being comfortable and trusting your hypnotherapist is essential. This is why it is advised that you take time to research hypnotherapists in your area and find out more about them, how they work and what their qualifications entail. You can arrange to meet with them before the procedure to ensure you feel comfortable with them.

Is Gastric Band Hypnosis Safe?

Gastric band hypnotic therapy is 100% safe. Your experienced hypnotherapist will only work with you to help you convince yourself that the decision to reduce food consumption, food types and change diet is a perfectly normal one. The only focal point of the therapy is to help the patient lose weight, reduce the size of their stomach and to increase self-confidence and feel far more positive about themselves.

What Are The Advantages Of Gastric Band Hypnotherapy Over Surgery?

The main advantage of gastric band hypnotherapy is that it allows a far more natural weight loss occurrence to take place. One thing all experts agree on is that drastic shifts in weight loss or weight gain are not good for the body and quite often with gastric band surgery, there is drastic weight loss. This puts unnecessary strain on the body's heart and other major organs.

Other Things To Consider Are:

- ❖ The substantial savings in the cost of the surgery, which can be upwards of £7,000
- ❖ No invasive surgery and associated recovery time
- ❖ No potential surgery complications
- ❖ Gastric band hypnosis helps train the mind about food, so manageable portions, reduction in fatty food consumption and sweet food consumption
- ❖ Promotes a healthy more positive and optimistic future

What Is Involved In Gastric Band Hypnosis?

Gastric band hypnosis is a session-based therapy, you wouldn't expect to be "cured" in a single session. We envisage 4-5 sessions have the best effect over a period. Remember most behavioral patterns, of which overeating and bad-diet are both, need to be "rained" out of our system. Gastric band hypnosis works with your subconscious mind to retrain underlying behavioral habits.

One thing you should consider is that whilst we average 4-5 sessions, each individual is different and the depth of therapy needed will vary. Once your hypnotherapist has assessed the issues and needs of the patient, and they have agreed to move forward with the treatment, a full case history is created for records purposes. Gastric band hypnotherapy also requires supporting activity and you would expect to be provided with either an MP3 or Cd that you can play to reinforce the subliminal suggestion.

Who Can Gastric Band Hypnotherapy Help?

Again, gastric band hypnotherapy is judged on a case by case basis, at my practice my clients typically are looking to lose 3 or more stone in weight (around 20 kg). However, a good hypnotherapist will judge each case based on a very in-depth assessment of suitability.

Hypnotherapy Supports Your Diet By:

- ❖ Planting subconscious suggestion
- ❖ Removing the need to cheat
- ❖ Learn why dieting doesn't change your habits
- ❖ Hypnosis has proven results in aiding weight loss.

Many people have to understand that a bad or unhealthy diet usually comes from years of habitual training in your food consumption.

Working late, lack of access to healthy, suitable alternatives, lifestyle and a lack of understanding of what's good and what isn't contribute. Hypnosis guide to why diets fail will help you understand these issues.

CHAPTER 6 - TIPS AND TRICKS FOR HYPNOSIS FOR WEIGHT LOSS

Weight Loss Hypnotists- Tips For Weight Loss

Among a long list of weight loss hypnotists in your area, find the best one for you with the help of this article so that you can lose weight for good with hypnosis.

1. Recommendations By Friends

If you get a recommendation for weight loss hypnotists from someone you know, great. But don't rely on their word alone. Ask them a few questions to find out more, for example:

- ❖ Was there a thorough consultation?
- ❖ Was the program adjusted to their individual needs?
- ❖ What was the most helpful thing the practitioner(s) did?
- ❖ Did the hypnotist(s) allow them to space their sessions out over some time?

2. Disregard All Advertising

I will always advise people to disregard advertising because advertising can be very misleading. You are much better advised to do your research. If you have no recommendations from anyone in your circle, make up a list of hypnotherapists in your area. You can find their contact details online or in local publications.

Research Them Online First: You might be able to establish their training and qualifications and professional memberships from that before you talk to them.

3. Training, Qualifications, Experience, And Membership Of Professional Associations

A good place to start your inquiry is with the basics. You want to know that the weight loss hypnotists you are considering have undergone solid training that involved case studies, that they hold a valid qualification (and license, depending on local regulations). You also want to make sure they adhere to the ethical standards of a professional body.

4. Talk To All Prospective Weight Loss Hypnotists On The Phone

Following up on your online research with phone calls to each weight loss hypnotist will take a little bit of effort. But seeing that you are about to invest a good chunk of money into your future, this effort will be worth it, I promise. One or two people will stand out from the crowd. Ask them the issue-specific questions below, but all the while also listens out for other things, for example:

- How is the hypnotist relating to you?
- Are they listening to your concerns?
- Are they personable?
- Are they accommodating?
- Are they professional?
- Do their answers to your questions make sense to you?

5. Beware Of Promises That Sound Too Good To Be True

I have heard of the odd unethical hypnotist who will promise quick weight loss through hypnosis. Beware. In reality, losing weight the natural way with hypnosis will take time. Your body and mind will both have to adjust step by step. This is not a bad thing, remember, you are changing your life rather than going for a quick fix. There are no overnight miracles, not even with a powerful therapy like hypnosis. One personal pet peeve of mine is the phrase 'I will make you lose weight'. This phrase implies that they will do all the work and you will have to do none. Well, even with a powerful therapy like hypnosis that is simply not how it works.

Expect To Take Responsibility: Nobody can MAKE you lose weight. A hypnotherapist can help you bring your subconscious mind on board with your weight loss plan, but you will have to put in some effort into making your weight loss plan become a reality.

6. Do They Have Any Other Qualification That Helps Them To Help Their Clients?

Hypnosis is a wonderful tool. It addresses the weight loss issue through the mind and changes your brain to embrace losing weight. If you want to improve on that and get the best possible treatment outcomes, check with the weight loss hypnotists on your list if they have any additional skills such as a coaching or psychotherapy qualification, a qualification as a dietician or nutritionist, or training in cognitive behavioral therapy (CBT). Additional skills can help you better integrate the changes you make during hypnotherapy sessions.

- They can help you establish new habits.
- They can help you gain a deeper understanding of your process.

In short, these additional skills can complement and greatly enhance your weight loss journey. Find out what the weight loss hypnotists on your list have to offer and don't be shy asking your questions.

7. Can I Spread My Program Over Time?

This is an important question to ask. Weight loss hypnosis can be costly. It is certainly more expensive than any of the standard weight loss programs. The way many clients make hypnosis affordable is by spreading out the work over some time. Hypnotherapy works very well this way and taking breaks between sessions makes sense anyway because your body and mind have a lot of adjusting to do as you are changing old habits and losing weight.

8. Can You Provide Me With A Maintenance Session I Can Use At Home?

Having a maintenance hypnosis recording to work with at home is particularly important when you spread the sessions over time. Listening to a weight loss hypnosis recording every day will keep you on track, to stay highly motivated and focused on your goal.

9. Can You Tailor Make A Weight Loss Hypnosis Program For Me?

There is research evidence that shows that individualized hypnosis treatments work better than generic ones. This makes a lot of sense because, of course, everyone is unique. Check with the weight loss hypnotists on your list if they are open to adjusting their program so it will be the exact right plan for you.

10. Does Your Program Start With An In-Depth Consultation?

Designing individualized programs for people, of course, will require an in-depth consultation at the start of your program, so make sure they provide this before ever working with hypnotherapy. I would say the first hour should be spent simply talking with you, establishing your needs, your concerns, finding out your history, what your issues and triggers are, how much weight you want to lose, any weight loss programs you have tried, etc. To me, it is a shame you should have to ask this question at all. An in-depth consultation should be a natural start to any treatment.

Unfortunately, however, not all weight loss hypnotists work in the same way. I have heard of some that simply place clients in a 'treatment' room listening to a hypnosis CD. (This, of course, helps them to 'treat' multiple clients at once.) I have heard of others who claim to 'make you lose weight' in less than 30 minutes, which also means there is no consultation involved. Unfortunately, these few bad apples make life hard for the solid core of the profession by giving it a bad reputation. So, to cut a long story short, do shop around. Make sure you will get a thorough consultation at the start of your program. The effort you put in at this stage will pay off in securing you to get the best service possible.

11. How Much Do You Charge Per Session?

Of course, you will need to check the cost of the program and the per-session cost.

Do Put That Cost In Context Though:

- ❖ Firstly, a thorough overview of how weight loss hypnosis compares to other weight loss programs and a delve into the benefits of weight loss by hypnosis may be helpful to understand what you are investing in by choosing hypnosis.
- ❖ Secondly, weigh up the cost involved against the quality of service you can expect based on your research.
- ❖ Thirdly, please don't look at the projected cost as a frivolous expenditure. Instead, view it as an investment in yourself. You do want to shift that weight issue and change your life after all, am I right?
- ❖ And, finally, do take into account that you can spread out your program over time which makes weight loss hypnosis much more affordable.

12. How Long Should Your Treatment Be?

This question should be left until the end of your consultation when your weight loss hypnotist has a good idea of your particular situation.

It would be hard for me to pin down what they may suggest because everybody works in different ways. All I can do here is give you some pointers as to factors to take into account in the design of your weight loss hypnosis program. Go over the set of 20 questions in my article 'Could you Lose Weight by Hypnosis?' to see where you are on the spectrum concerning your weight issue- on the conscious eating side, or the emotional eating side. My rule of thumb is that the more weight you want to lose, and the more you identify with the 'emotional eating' side of the spectrum, the longer you must plan for your weight loss hypnosis program. If you identify as an emotional eater, your issues very likely started early in life. Therefore, if you find yourself on the emotional eating side of the spectrum, you will also be alerted to the necessity to do some regression work to look at food issues originating in your childhood. If this sounds far-fetched to you, to find out what these issues may be, please check my article 'Could you Lose Weight by Hypnosis?' which goes into detail on this topic.

Top Ten Ways To Lose Weight

Whilst it is important to ensure that you're not overweight and equally important to lead a healthy lifestyle, you certainly don't want to get into bad weight loss habits, so deciphering the good advice from the bad is important.

The first thing you should do before starting any form of weight loss program is to consult your doctor about the method of weight loss you are interested in. Your doctor can give you helpful advice and also perhaps give you a medical check to ensure that any program you do start doesn't harm your health. The following top-ten methods listed in this article are not suggested methods, instead, this article aims to provide you with the information at hand to decide which methods are right for you and which method you should avoid. Weight is a very personal subject and some of the techniques listed in this article are for those people who are classed as morbidly obese and are not necessarily suitable for those who are just a little overweight. Again, getting a professional medical assessment is critical to your long term health and weight loss success.

Discover Our Top Ten Ways To Lose Weight:

1) Start To Exercise More

When you think about how you can lose weight, you generally think of two methods, the first is dieting and the second is exercising. Starting an exercise regime can be daunting for anyone who hasn't been interested in doing sport much. When you're overweight it can be even harder to motivate yourself to start. Joining a gym can be a good method to motivate you to train, as the cost of the gym membership going out of your bank account every month can hurt the wallet if you are simply wasting the money! This can be motivation enough to pack your gym bag. Another reason to join a gym is that they are a good place to get professional advice on exercising. Most mainstream gyms have Personal Trainers who can help and advise you and also design a fitness program that meets your needs. Generally, these fitness programs are then assessed every few months to check on your progress.

The trick to keeping up any exercise routine is to set yourself realistic goals or challenges so that you will always having something to work towards, also it is important to keep the exercise fun. When training and fitness become a chore it is very easy for your subconscious to come up with any number of reasons not to exercise. As soon as you start skipping exercise sessions it becomes much easier not to stick to your plan.

2) Weight Loss Medication

The thought that you can take a pill to help you lose weight sounds fantastic in principle seemingly providing you with a 'magical' solution to your weight problems. However, for many people who decide to use weight loss medication the risks and potential side effects can outweigh the benefits.

Without discussing the merits or disadvantages of particular brands it is important to consider that there could be side effects from taking these medications so doing so should only be carried out once medical advice is sort. Although this form of medication is freely available to buy from the Internet it is advisable to only take these medicines if they have been specifically prescribed by a doctor to treat your obesity condition as not only could you waste money on the unnecessary medication you could be seriously risking your health.

3) Go On A Diet

The thought of going on a diet horrifies some people, but there normally comes a point when a person decides enough is enough they have to lose weight, therefore they must go on a diet! Does the question then become what diet to choose? There are hundreds if not thousands of different diet plans out on the market some much healthier than others, and some downright dangerous to your health. No matter what diet you choose to go on there are some fundamental principles that you could consider when trying to lose weight by dieting. Firstly, calories are offset by calories out. What this means is the fundamental thing controlling your weight is the number of calories that you consume through eating and the number of calories you use by either exercising or going about your daily life.

Typically a woman should consume 2,000 calories a day and a man 2,500 (although these are average figures). By reducing your calorie intake below these figures should, in theory, allow you to lose weight. However, there is something else to consider and that is your metabolism. If you drastically reduce your calorie intake then your body can go into something called 'starvation mode' which effectively slows down weight loss as your body tries to 'hold on' to its fat stores. For someone who is trying to lose weight, this defeats the purpose. So the solution is to only reduce your calorie intake enough so that you lose a little weight, for example, 1 pound per week is a sensible target which is achievable without starving yourself and more importantly it allows you to subtly change your diet to compensate for this, making it much easier in the long term to maintain the weight loss.

Nutrition is also an important thing to consider when picking a diet. You should aim to eat a healthy, nutritious diet which ultimately is well balanced. A well-balanced diet is a diet that includes food from the five main food groups (but reducing Fat and Sugar), which are:

- ❖ Meat, Fish, and Alternatives (Eggs, Beans, Pulses)
- ❖ Bread, Cereals, and Potatoes
- ❖ Fruit and Vegetables
- ❖ Milk and Dairy Produce
- ❖ Fat and Sugar

Any diet that is rich in fruit or vegetables is likely to be a healthy one. You don't have to skip eating foods with fat and sugar. However, you should be looking to reduce your intake in this area as we generally eat way too much from this particular food group.

4) Gastric Bands

A gastric band is a bariatric surgical procedure where a band is placed around the top of the stomach making it smaller in size so that the stomach fills up with food quicker than it would under normal circumstances. Gastric band (or Lap-Band) surgery is a fairly drastic procedure best suited to those who are classed as obese on the BMI scale. Whilst there are potential complications and risks associated with any surgery the benefits can include a great deal of weight loss in some situations a person can lose up to 60% of their body weight. For those who are obese and have constantly struggled with their weight loss then gastric band surgery can help. As bariatric surgery is not necessarily the preferred method for all individuals this method should be fully discussed with a professional to get a firm understanding of both the benefits and risks of undertaking gastric band surgery.

5) Gastric Balloons

A gastric balloon is a silicone balloon that is placed inside a person's stomach and filled with saline. This balloon then makes a person feel as though they are full up, making them less inclined to eat, forcing a person to eat smaller portions. The gastric balloon is inserted into a person's stomach using a fairly simple procedure- basically passing the balloon through the mouth, down the throat, and into the stomach.

The balloon is then filled and left to float freely in the stomach.

6) Eat Less & Drink More Water

Probably the simplest way to lose weight is to just eat less than you normally eat. Perhaps this means reducing portion size or making slight changes to your diet, such as not having second helpings of your favorite dessert, but eating less regularly will help you lose weight. Substituting certain foods with other foods can help reduce calories and help you to lose weight. For example, if you have a ham sandwich with full-fat mayonnaise for lunch, substituting the ham for turkey, and full-fat mayonnaise for low-fat mayonnaise can save you a lot of calories, whilst not compromising the taste of your lunch!

7) Go For A Walk

If you hate dieting and also hate the thought of having to go to the gym then you could consider going for a walk regularly. Depending on how much you weigh and how fast you walk, you could burn off around 100 calories per mile that you walk. This may not sound like much but an hour a day walking could help you burn an additional 700 calories a week or the equivalent of a normal-sized meal!

8) Hypnosis

Hypnosis is a state of concentration and relaxation where a patient enters an enhanced state of awareness allowing a hypnotherapist to suggest ideas and lifestyle changes to the patient. Hypnosis aims to re-program patterns of behavior within the mind. Hypnosis can help you lose weight by allowing you to develop a new self-image whilst also teaching you to be more relaxed about your weight loss (stress can lead to comfort eating). You can find a hypnotherapist who can treat you directly or you can even find hypnotherapy CDs and programs online that are much cheaper than visiting a consultant.

9) Psychological Triggers

As fully committed to a diet or exercise plan that you are, sometimes your 'mind' can get the better of you. It's natural to think that when you're on a 'diet' you are somehow depriving yourself and making a sacrifice. These psychological 'sacrifices' can be difficult to maintain constantly. Perhaps you've had a bad day and your will power is wavering. Therefore it is a good idea to implement some psychological techniques to help you make positive diet and exercise choices. Their following tips can help you lose weight whilst bolstering your weight loss intentions:

- ❖ Use smaller plates- putting your food onto a smaller plate tricks your brain into thinking you're eating a bigger portion
- ❖ Don't feel like exercising? Tell yourself to change into your gym clothes first and then decided. Sometimes once you're changed you feel much more ready to exercise.
- ❖ Don't cut out everything you love from your diet. Love chocolate? Try eating a couple of pieces once or twice a week as a treat instead of a bar a night! You'll soon come to appreciate the smaller piece more and you'll feel better if you start to lose some weight!

Remember there are many ways you can lose weight and by using psychological techniques this gives you another method to employ from your weight-loss arsenal.

10) Get A Tummy Tuck

For some people, it can be almost impossible to lose excess weight in certain areas. For those who have already lost a great deal of weight or have had a baby, it is possible to have a lot of loose skin around the abdomen area. This loose skin can be difficult to shift through traditional dieting or exercising. In these instances, the cosmetic surgery procedure called abdominoplasty or tummy tuck could be used. A tummy tuck is a cosmetic surgery procedure that is implemented to help make the abdomen area much firmer.

When excess skin and fat from the abdomen area are removed this tightens the muscle of the abdominal wall.

Weight Loss By Hypnosis- 7 Huge Benefits

In this article, I have compiled the most prominent benefits of weight loss through hypnosis so that you may get an idea if you may want to give the treatment a go.

1. No Weigh-Ins

Many of my weight loss clients have told me about negative experiences with other weight loss programs that used weigh-ins as a means of trying to motivate participants to lose weight. Often, stepping on the scales in front of a group can have the opposite effect to what program leaders intend. Weight loss clients have often been struggling with their weight issues for quite some time, and are acutely aware that they are overweight. Many may weigh themselves at home regularly if not obsessively in an attempt to gain control over the situation. Pointing out their exact weight to them in front of a group can, therefore, be a shaming experience rather than an encouraging one. This holds especially if it is hard for them to follow the program at the prescribed pace. Weight loss by hypnosis does not use weigh-ins. In the hypnosis world, we don't believe weight loss is about the exact numbers. Rather, it is about an overall goal to re-gain control and to change direction in your life at your own pace while allowing you to keep your privacy about your exact weight.

2. No Calorie Counting, No Prescribed Diet Plans

Many weight loss clients who have tried other weight loss programs before they came for hypnosis describe feeling under pressure by diet plans and calorie counting. Some describe that they were not able to stick to that prescribed plan and ended up falling behind, resulting ultimately in feelings of shame and failure. With weight loss by hypnosis, there is no counting of calories. There are no prescribed targets or diet plans, instead, you are encouraged to put your plan and targets in place. The basic underlying premise in weight loss hypnosis is that your mind plays a very big role in the weight loss process. Therefore, your mind is supported in coming back to healthy eating patterns that sustain you, and at the same time allow excess weight to fall off.

What Do Those Individual Weight Loss Plans Look Like? People Do This In Different Ways:.

- ❖ Some people decide to educate their mind through hypnosis to eat more consciously. This means to chew slowly, to notice the body's signals as to when you are full and as a result they find themselves eating smaller portions.
- ❖ Other people decide on dietary changes- for example substituting processed foods with fruit and veg.

- ❖ Some people decide to educate their mind to ditch all sugar.
- ❖ The choices people make will depend on how much weight they want to lose and on their personal preferences.

3. Hypnosis Caters For Individual Differences

Every hypnosis weight loss client is an individual with different needs, wants and preferences. The weight loss solution looks slightly different for each person. Being treated as an individual leaves you the independence to lose weight at your own pace, the freedom to eat what you decide to eat and to make your unique plan as to what is right for you to do to lose weight.

4. Weight Loss By Hypnosis Does Not Rely On Weight Loss Products

Clients who have attended other weight loss programs before hypnosis often talks to me about weight loss products that some other programs rely on. More often than not their experience is that a dependency on the product is being set up. While they use the product, they do experience some weight loss and once they stop using it, they gain weight quite quickly and then they are back where they started. Some even gain more weight than they had previously. There are no weight loss products involved in weight loss by hypnosis. Here, you can lose weight naturally, and at your own pace. This is an important benefit to you because it brings out your internal resources for losing weight and step by step you will learn that 'you can do this', resulting in feelings of confidence and self-worth.

5. Motivation And Determination

Have you ever dieted and felt a sense of loss when you couldn't eat x, y or z? Have you ever felt resentment because your partner or friend could eat x, y or z? Or, have you felt like a true martyr when it felt that your weight loss plan caused you to experience hardship?, When that happens, you are in a place of lack where you, very quickly, lose motivation and, in turn, determination to see your weight loss plan through. Many clients fail at that point. Think about it. As long as you feel you are missing out on something or that you would rather do something else, following your weight loss plan is very hard.

In contrast, weight loss by hypnosis works through your mind and helps you to instill one important piece that many weight loss programs fail to instill- a genuine deep desire to lose weight. This desire automatically results in strong motivation and determination to do whatever you have to do to see your weight loss goals. Weight loss by hypnosis makes working towards your goal easy. By working on your mind, it creates a situation where you will want to follow your plan, and where you will feel good about following your plan. You can then enjoy getting results, and that, in turn, will boost the desire to keep going.

6. Weight Loss By Hypnosis Is Weight Loss Made Easy

When planning to lose weight, your first port of call is usually losing weight through willpower- setting up a diet plan and enforcing that plan every day- fighting against cravings, fighting against a growing sense of resentment. Willpower usually will only last so long. After a bit of a struggle, many people give up and go back to their old eating habits because pushing through is just too hard. With weight loss by hypnosis, you are bringing your mind and emotions, both, on board with the process. You will experience a reduction in food cravings along with a sense of purpose that losing weight is your number one goal.

In this way, weight loss by hypnosis can take the mental struggle out of the weight loss process.

- ❖ No more giving into cravings and feeling ashamed afterward.
- ❖ No more struggle followed by a sense of failure.

Instead, losing weight happens almost without you noticing it, almost playfully, without any 'efforting' involved- very easily indeed. Imagine how much easier things could be without that constant mental struggle, and negative feelings constantly bothering you, resulting in you feeling bad about yourself. If you temporarily experience a glitch and fall back onto some old habits, weight loss by hypnosis encourages you to go easy on yourself and to simply go back to your plan and continue as if nothing ever happened. No more giving up because you made one 'mistake'. Instead, we recognize that the weight loss journey is a process that does take some time and involves learning experiences.

In this way, with weight loss hypnosis, you are sort of 'getting out of your own way', putting a stop to the struggle, so that you are then able to 'just get on' with your weight loss plan.

7. Weight Loss By Hypnosis Works For Permanent Change

Many weight loss clients who have experienced other weight loss programs are used to a quick-fix approach. Most programs count pounds, count calories, and if you have met your target at the end of the program you are deemed to be a success story. Well, some people are and some are not. Many people will regain the weight they lost quite quickly after the program ends. This is because their mind and emotions are in the same place they were before the weight loss program.

As A Result:

- ❖ The same cravings are likely to kick in.
- ❖ The same mental struggle can occupy the mind.
- ❖ The same habits might well win over.

In Contrast:

- ❖ Weight loss by hypnosis is not a quick fix.
- ❖ Weight loss hypnosis is not a miracle cure.
- ❖ Instead, weight loss hypnosis has a goal of working towards permanent change.

This weight loss journey is not just about you losing x-amount of pounds. It's about you gaining the weight, size, and shape that is right for your unique body, and it is about being able to hold on to those changes in the long run.

Weight loss by hypnosis is also about you being happy with your body and feeling good about yourself. Because at the end of the day, life is about more than your weight. It is about enjoying your own very unique body and changing your life so that you can be happy with who you are.

CHAPTER 7 - BINGE EATING SUPPRESSION

Binge Eating

Binge eating is a pattern of disordered eating which consists of episodes of uncontrollable eating. It is a common symptom of eating disorders such as binge eating disorder and bulimia nervosa. During such binges, a person rapidly consumes an excessive quantity of food. A diagnosis of binge eating is associated with feelings of loss of control.

Causes Of Bing Eating

There are no direct causes of binge eating; however, long term dieting, psychological issues, and an obsession with body image have been linked to binge eating. Multiple factors increase a person's risk of developing binge eating disorder. Family history can play a role if you have had someone in your family who was affected by binge eating. A person may not have a supportive or friendly home environment and they have a hard time expressing their problems of BED. Having a history of going on extreme diets may cause an urge to binge eat. Psychological issues such as feeling negative about yourself or the way you look may trigger a bing

Treatments Of Binge Eating

There are many ways to treat binge eating disorder mainly through different types of therapy. There is Behavioral Weight Loss therapy (BWL) that is meant to help a person make gradual lifestyle changes to their diet and eating habits. Cognitive Behavioral Therapy (CBT) targets the chaotic eating habits of a person with BED and encourages a regular meal plan. Interpersonal Psychotherapy (IPT) addresses the social deficits of BED and promotes lifestyle changes. Dialectical Behavioral Therapy (DBT) is used to teach healthy ways of dealing with emotional arousals or urges

Symptoms Of Binge Eating

Most people with binge-eating disorder are overweight or obese, but you may be at a normal weight. Behavioral and emotional signs and symptoms of binge-eating disorder include:

- Eating unusually large amounts of food in a specific amount of time, such as over two hours
- Feeling that your eating behavior is out of control
- Eating even when you're full or not hungry
- Eating rapidly during binge episodes
- Eating until you're uncomfortably full
- Frequently eating alone or in secret
- Feeling depressed, disgusted, ashamed, guilty or upset about your eating

- ❖ Frequently dieting, possibly without weight loss

Unlike a person with bulimia, after a binge, you don't regularly compensate for extra calories eaten by vomiting, using laxatives or exercising excessively. You may try to diet or eat normal meals. But restricting your diet may simply lead to more binge eating. The severity of the binge-eating disorder is determined by how often episodes of bingeing occur during a week.

Health Risks Of Binge Eating

There are several physicals, emotional, and social health risks when one is suffering from Binge Eating Disorder (BED). Amongst the health risks is the running chance of extreme weight gain. This problem results in two-thirds of those with the disorder to become overweight or obese. With obesity comes a myriad of health complications. Some of them being:

- ❖ Sleep Apnea
- ❖ Cancer
- ❖ Heart Disease
- ❖ High Blood Pressure
- ❖ Type 2 Diabetes
- ❖ Arthritis

Effects Of Binge Eating

Typically the eating is done rapidly and a person will feel emotionally numb and unable to stop eating. Most people who have eating binges try to hide this behavior from others and often feel ashamed about being overweight or depressed about their overeating. Although people who do not have an eating disorder may occasionally experience episodes of overeating, frequent binge eating is often a symptom of an eating disorder.

Binge-eating disorder, as the name implies, is characterized by uncontrollable, excessive eating, followed by feelings of shame and guilt. Unlike those with bulimia, those with binge-eating disorder symptoms typically do not purge their food, fast, or excessively exercise to compensate for binges. Additionally, these individuals tend to diet more often, enroll in weight-control programs and have a history of family obesity. However, many who have bulimia also have binge-eating disorder.

Along with the social and physical health that is affected when suffering from Binge Eating Disorder (BED), there are psychiatric disorders that are often linked to BED. Some of them being, but are not limited to:

- ❖ Depression
- ❖ Bipolar Disorder
- ❖ Anxiety Disorder
- ❖ Substance Abuse/Use Disorder

Binge Eating: Keeping A Healthy Weight

If you have binge eating disorder, getting well needs to be your No. 1 priority. You'll first need counseling to find out why you are overeating and how to stop. When your bingeing stops, you'll probably lose weight. Keeping that weight off -- and reaching a healthy weight -- is important for your overall health. That can be hard for anyone, but it may be especially tricky for binge eaters. You'll want to work with your doctors and a dietitian to make sure you don't have a setback. "You want to establish a healthy eating pattern and not slip into dieting, which could set up the next round of bingeing,

What Is Weight Suppression And Why Is It A Problem?

Weight suppression is the difference between one's highest adult body weight and one's current weight. It can also be thought of as the amount of weight one has lost from a previous high weight, usually in response to dieting. Human bodies are meant to be a variety of shapes and sizes. When a person who is genetically programmed to be in a larger body tries to reduce his or her size to smaller than intended by genetics, binge eating may be the body's natural defense to avoid death by starvation and return the body to a healthier size for that body. Weight loss, even among healthy people, decreases metabolism and the amount of energy the body burns. It also seems to increase appetite. The hormone leptin, which sends satiety signals to the brain, is believed to play a role in this process. Studies indicate that individuals with high weight suppression appear to have reduced levels of leptin. For these reasons, there is a strong biological predisposition to regain lost weight.

How To Know If Your Weight Is Suppressed

Some questions to consider:

- ❖ Is your weight lower than your highest adult weight?
- ❖ Are you preoccupied with thoughts about food?
- ❖ Do you experience episodes of eating in which you eat unusually large amounts of food in a short period and feel out of control while doing so?
- ❖ Do you eat impulsively–when you haven't planned to– or engage in emotional eating?

If more than one of the above is true, consider seeking help and gaining weight. Getting to a weight that is biologically determined healthy for you, regardless of where that number is on population norms, is usually the healthiest. We do not yet have enough research to know whether you would need to go back to your highest weight, or whether regaining some of the suppressed weight may be sufficient. You may find that weight gain will relieve some preoccupation with food, reduce symptoms of bulimia nervosa, and generally improve the quality of your life. You may also discover that the negative consequences of weight gain that you fear do not materialize.

Why Do I Binge Eat? And How Do I Stop?

Binge eating can affect your quality of life, your sense of well-being and your health. However, it can be difficult to stop binge eating, despite the negative health effects. Fortunately, by learning helpful coping strategies and identifying the psychological reasons you binge eat, you can begin to work to overcome them.

Binge Eating vs Overeating

Before exploring why you binge eat, it's useful to have a general understanding of what binge eating is and how it's different from overeating. Binge eating disorder is characterized by repeated episodes of eating more in a specific period than most people would under similar circumstances. There is often a feeling of loss of control that comes with binge eating.

Binge eating disorder typically also involves:

- ❖ Feelings of disgust, guilt or embarrassment directed toward oneself
- ❖ Eating alone to conceal the behavior
- ❖ Episodes that occur at least once a week for three months

❖ Significant distress after bingeing

Unlike binge eating, overeating tends not to happen recurrently or be driven by a sense of lack of control. In most cases, overeating also does not trigger the same intense feelings of guilt and shame that binge eating does.

5 Reasons People Binge Eat

The reasons people binge eat can vary from person-to-person. However, there are some general patterns people tend to follow if they struggle with binge eating or a diagnosed binge eating disorder.

1. Genetics

Is binge eating disorder genetic? It's possible that binge eating disorder is genetic or at least partially connected to certain genetic risk factors. The same genetic risk factors linked to binge eating disorder are also associated with an increased risk of substance use disorders and other eating disorders. In a recent study from the Boston University School of Medicine, researchers identified one gene that was connected to binge eating in mice.

2. Depression

Depression and binge eating disorder are often closely linked. However, it can be a challenge to know which causes the other. For example, someone might binge eat because they're depressed, or their binge eating may cause symptoms of depression.

3. Low Self-Esteem

Self-esteem, body image, and eating disorders are all often closely linked to one another. In many cases, low self-esteem or poor body image trigger feelings of guilt and shame that people cope with by binge eating. Conversely, the feelings of guilt and shame that many people experience after binge eating can lead to worsened self-esteem and body image.

4. Stress And Anxiety

Stress is a common trigger for binge eating. Many people use eating as a coping mechanism to deal with stress or anxiety.

5. Dieting

It may seem counterintuitive, but many people begin binge-eating after dieting. People dieting sometimes control their food intake to the point that they have intense cravings for food. As a response, many of these people binge eat. Slipping up on a diet can also lead to feelings of guilt, which can trigger binge eating.

How To Overcome Binge Eating

Learning how to stop binge eating isn't easy, but it's certainly possible. Overcoming binge eating often relies on identifying triggers and reasons for bingeing. Once you recognize the reasons you're binge eating, you can start to find specific methods to help you control binge eating.

The following strategies can help you combat the urge to binge eat:

1. **Keep A Food Diary:** A food diary can help you be more mindful of what you're eating and make it easier to identify triggers. It can also serve as a place to keep track of your moods and feelings.
2. **Plan Out Your Meals:** Meal planning can help you develop eating healthier patterns, and make it easier to control what you eat. As part of a binge eating meal plan prevention strategy, ensure that you have the ingredients you need to make everything on your meal plan. This cuts out the uncertainty or instability that may be a trigger for binge eating.
3. **Portion Out Your Food:** Much like meal planning, food portion control can help you take more control over your eating habits and reduce the chance that you'll fall back into a binge eating pattern. Removing extra junk food from your kitchen and sticking with weekly shopping, meal planning, and portion control routine can help set you up for success.

4. **Don't Eat Alone:** One of the primary signs of binge eating disorder is feeling ashamed or embarrassed about your eating habits, which can lead you to binge eat when alone. Improve accountability and reduce negative patterns by always trying to eat meals with another person.

5. **Avoid Yo-Yo Dieting:** Yo-yo dieting is a vicious cycle of weight loss and weight gain. Not only can it increase the likelihood of binge eating, but it's also an unhealthy and unsustainable way to lose weight or maintain a healthy weight. Focus more on developing sustainable, long-term healthy eating habits rather than trying extreme deprivation or fad diets.

6. **Seek Support:** Binge eating disorder can feel like something that takes over your life. You may require additional help and professional support. Fortunately, different options are available for treating binge eating disorder, including therapy. Therapy can help you develop healthy coping mechanisms. You may also find benefit in a binge eating support group, as social support can be invaluable when you're dealing with an eating disorder.

CHAPTER 8 - INSTRUCTIONS TO ENSURE THAT MEDITATION FOR WEIGHT LOSS

What Is Meditation?

Meditation is a practice that helps to connect the mind and body to achieve a sense of calm. People have been meditating for thousands of years as a spiritual practice. Today, many people use meditation to reduce stress and become more aware of their thoughts. Meditation is simply the act of focusing your attention to become more mindful. The American Meditation Society explains that "during meditation, the attention flows inward instead of engaging in the outside world of activity." According to the organization, a meditation practice can awaken positive qualities in you.

There are many types of meditation. Some are based on the use of specific phrases called mantras. Others focus on breathing or keeping the mind in the present moment. All of these methods can help you develop a better understanding of yourself, including how you mind and bodywork. This increased awareness makes meditation a useful tool for better understanding your eating habits, which could result in weight loss. Read on to learn more about the benefits of meditation for weight loss and how to get started.

What Are The Benefits Of Meditation For Weight Loss?

Meditation won't make you lose weight overnight. But with a little practice, it can potentially have lasting effects on not only your weight but also your thought patterns.

Sustainable Weight Loss

Meditation is linked to a variety of benefits. In terms of weight loss, mindfulness meditation seems to be the most helpful. A 2017 review of existing studies found that mindfulness meditation was an effective method for losing weight and changing eating habits.

Mindfulness Meditation Involves Paying Close Attention To:

- ❖ Where you are
- ❖ What you're doing
- ❖ How you're feeling in the present moment

During mindfulness meditation, you'll acknowledge all of these aspects without judgment. Try to treat your actions and thoughts as just those — nothing else. Take stock of what you're feeling and doing, but try not to classify anything as being good or bad. This becomes easier with regular practice.

Practicing mindfulness meditation can lead to long-term benefits, too. Compared to other dieters, those practicing mindfulness are more likely to keep the weight off.

Less Guilt And Shame

Mindfulness meditation can be particularly helpful in curbing emotional and stress-related eating. By becoming more aware of your thoughts and emotions, you can recognize those times when you eat because you're stressed, rather than hungry. It's also a good tool to prevent you from falling into the harmful spiral of shame and guilt that some people fall into when trying to change their eating habits. Mindfulness meditation involves recognizing your feelings and behaviors for what they are, without judging yourself.

This encourages you to forgive yourself for making mistakes, such as stress-eating a bag of potato chips. That forgiveness can also prevent you from catastrophizing, which is a fancy term for what happens when you decide to order a pizza since you already "screwed up" by eating a bag of chips.

Meditation For Weight Loss

Scientists have studied the effects of meditation on our bodies and have found that the practice can help us to relax, sleep better and improve our health. But they are also beginning to explore how meditation can help us lose weight. In one recent research review, scientists evaluated the role of how meditation can affect weight loss and certain behaviors that are often linked to poor eating. They found that mindful meditation can help to decrease the frequency of emotional eating and binge eating. Other studies have also found that using stress reduction techniques, like meditation, can have a positive impact on results during a weight loss program. Of course, researchers can't say that meditation alone will make you lose weight. But since the practice of meditation is free, carries no side effects and provides other health benefits, why not use it to help you curb emotional eating and create more mindful food habits?

How Can I Start Meditating For Weight Loss?

Anyone with a mind and body can practice meditation. There's no need for any special equipment or expensive classes. For many, the hardest part is simply finding the time. Try to start with something reasonable, such as 10 minutes a day or even every other day. Make sure you have access to a quiet place during these 10 minutes. If you have children, you may want to squeeze it in before they wake up or after they go to bed to minimize distraction. You can even try doing it in the shower.

Once you're in a quiet place, make yourself comfortable. You can sit or lie down in any position that feels easy. Start by focusing on your breath, watching your chest or stomach as it rises and falls. Feel the air as it moves in and out of your mouth or nose. Listen to the sounds the air makes. Do this for a minute or two, until you start to feel more relaxed.

Next, With Your Eyes Open Or Closed, Follow These Steps:

- ❖ Take a deep breath in. Hold it for several seconds.
- ❖ Slowly exhale and repeat.
- ❖ Breathe naturally.
- ❖ Observe your breath as it enters your nostrils, raises your chest, or moves your belly, but don't alter it in any way.
- ❖ Continue focusing on your breath for 5 to 10 minutes.
- ❖ You'll find your mind wandering, which is completely normal. Just acknowledge that your mind has wandered and returned your attention to your breath.
- ❖ As you start to wrap up, reflect on how easily your mind wandered. Then, acknowledge how easy it was to bring your attention back to your breath.

Try to do these more days of the week than not. Keep in mind that it might not feel very effective the first few times you do it. But with regular practice, it'll get easier and start to feel more natural.

How Can Meditation Help You Lose Weight?

Meditation is a powerful tool that can align the subconscious mind with the conscious mind to comply with changes we want in our behavior. It could be anything from controlling your food cravings and wanting to be more active, to simply reducing stress in one's life. Simply finding 20 minutes a day to meditate can help train your mind towards achieving a fitter body. Here's how meditation and weight loss are linked:

1. Meditation Heightens Your Awareness

Meditation helps in improving mental acuity and increases our awareness about ourselves. It enables the mind to slow down and focus more on things that matter and require attention.

2. It Helps Control Food Cravings

Focusing your mind to achieve goals can be done through meditation. The powerful concentration that is created due to meditation helps train the mind to be disenchanted by certain foods, cravings, and binge eating. The mind can also be focused on picturing a thinner self or a more active lifestyle, to align the subconscious and the conscious to act simultaneously. By changing desire at the root level, you can train the mind to eliminate certain foods and even replace them with healthier options.

3. Meditation Works To Reduce Stress

Stress is the leading cause of all ailments. It is one of the biggest reasons for weight gain as well. The body's coping mechanism makes it put on weight as a supposed defense against undesirable situations and outcomes. This is the primitive part of our body's functioning, where fat was piled on to fight the cold, hunger, and other stressful situations during the days of the 'early-man'. Reducing stress through meditation techniques can calm the mind and improve mental balance.

4. It Induces Better Assimilation Of Food

Meditation is a way of improving food assimilation in the body. Breaking down of nutrients and then absorbing them in the right way for bodily functions, can be improved through meditative techniques. By reducing stress, meditation also prevents broken down food to be stored as fat by utilizing it in the right way.

5. It Reduces Basal Metabolic Rate

Our Basal Metabolic rate or BMR is the quantity of energy expended in calories to maintain bodily functions. This has a profound effect on weight loss because a higher BMR means faster calorie burning. Practicing pranayama or meditation increases BMR and improves the body's metabolism. This will help manage your weight loss program in a better way.

Where Can I Find Guided Meditations?

if you're curious about trying other types of meditation or just want some guidance, you can find a variety of guided meditations online. Keep in mind that you don't necessarily need to follow one that's designed for weight loss. When choosing a guided meditation online, try to stay away from those promising overnight results or offering hypnosis.

Other Mindfulness Techniques

Here are a few other tips to help you take a mindfulness-based approach to weight loss:

- **Slow Down Your Meals:** Focus on chewing slowly and recognizing the taste of each bite.
- **Find The Right Time To Eat:** Avoid eating on the go or while multitasking.
- **Learn To Recognize Hunger And Fullness:** If you aren't hungry, don't eat. If you're full, don't keep going. Try to listen to what your body is telling you.
- **Recognize How Certain Foods Make You Feel:** Try to pay attention to how you feel after eating certain foods. Which ones make you feel tired? Which ones make you feel energized?
- **Forgive Yourself:** You thought that pint of ice cream would make you feel better, but it didn't. That's OK. Learn from it and move on.

- **Make More Thoughtful Food Choices:** Spend more time thinking about what you're going to eat before actually eating.
- **Notice Your Cravings:** Craving chocolate again? Acknowledging your cravings can help you resist them.

Other Points To Keep In Mind

A few other things to remember while performing yoga meditation for weight loss are:

- Be patient, as weight loss is a lengthy process that needs time and persistence.
- Have realistic expectations while you visualize your goals.
- Be honest with yourself about your cravings, likes, dislikes, and what you know you can surely do.
- Don't let negative thoughts fill your mind while you're focused.

CHAPTER 9 - DEVELOPING A POSITIVE ATTITUDE WITH SELF-HYPNOSIS

Think positively! You have probably heard this so many times that the phrase has lost its meaning. But having a positive attitude does not mean that you have to be happy, no matter what. It is about paying attention to what is happening around you and to react appropriately. A positive attitude is what spurs people into action. Being a positive person means being capable of planning, taking action, of remedying things that do not work. Opposed to that is a negative attitude – the type of thinking that prevents you from getting involved, from taking action, from finding solutions to the things that make you feel unhappy.

Discover What Makes You Happy

People tend to be unhappy because they do not do what they want to do. What is even more worrying, is that they no longer know what they want, and fail to even question what they want. People can get stuck in a routine without realizing that in time, they have created a prison around them that does not allow them to grow, to expand, to experiment and live their dreams. If you are unhappy with how your life is then you need to change something about it! It doesn't always need to be something of great importance, such as a new job or a new direction in life. You can focus on the little things too. As long as the changes make you happy, you will be on the right path. Thinking positively is actually about understanding life, including the good and the bad. Rediscover the importance of wanting things for yourself, things that make you happy. Find solutions and act when the situation requires such behavior. One big mistake that people often make is they compare themselves with other people who appear more successful, have more money, are more attractive, and so on. Such comparisons only breed envy and other similarly negative feelings. If you find yourself constantly comparing yourself to others, stop now! Keep this in mind. You are not inferior, even if other people try to make you feel this way. You are who you are. Discover what makes you happy!

Develop Positive Habits

We all experience the world through our five senses, what we see, what we hear, what we feel, what we smell, and what we say (to others and our self-talk). In any given situation, whether it's a walk in the park, sharing time with family or reading a good book, we are constantly taking on board more information from all five senses. So, why not do it constructively and choose just what you take on board? Below is a list of five questions I recommend you ask yourself every day. Write them down and put the list on your fridge door. You could even write the answer next to the questions each time you do it so you can look back and remember the positive feelings.

- ❖ What did I see that made me feel happy today?
- ❖ What did I enjoy the taste of today?
- ❖ What uplifting smell did I inhale today?
- ❖ What interesting sound(s) did I take in and enjoy today?
- ❖ What was it I touched that made me feel pleasure today?

Nothing succeeds like the success we see, feel, hear, smell and say. It is true, so why not learn from it? Positive thoughts breed positive actions. There is a positive spin to be found on just about everything. Sometimes it is hard to find it. We may have to search for it, but it is usually there. If we get in the habit of finding it and filling our lives with more positives then we will be healthier, happier, and achieve more.

Focus On The Positive

Words have power and this is certainly true when it comes to hypnosis. Within the framework of hypnotherapy, we almost always have to focus on the positive. It's much better when the words paint a picture of what is wanted, rather than of what isn't wanted. Which of these is better; "Every day I feel better and better" or "Every day I feel less depressed"? Using positive suggestions in self-hypnosis is about concentrating on what you want. It's about focusing on what's good for you. It's about focusing your energy in the right way. The words we use to bring up emotions and pictures in our mind and it's important that they are not only clear (to avoid ambiguity) but that they are framed in the positive. This keeps the focus on what you want. When we say, "I'm not going to get angry" well, then we're keeping the focus on anger. Simply saying, "I'm going to be calm" will help you to accomplish just that. Whether it is within self-hypnosis or in your everyday life, keeping your self-talk positive will help you achieve the results you desire. Focus on the positives, on solutions, on thinking in the right manner – so that things happen the way you want them to. Listening regularly to our self-hypnosis recordings can start to shape your thinking patterns, getting them closer to what you want for yourself.

Everyone Can Benefit

We can all benefit from developing a more positive outlook on life. When you do something well, allow yourself to feel pleased about it – even if it is just a small thing. By doing this you are nourishing yourself in the most practical way possible. And the more you expect positive things to happen in your life, the more they will. Positive thinking is a positive habit – the more you practice, the better you become. Positive habits become positive expectations. Take a moment and ask yourself; "Do I have the proper attitude towards life and myself?" If the answer is 'no', then it is time to begin your journey towards developing a newer, more positive you.

7 Positive Thinking Tips

Do you need some positive thinking tips to stay upbeat? Let's face it - there are a lot of reasons in this world to think negatively. And if you're walking around with "happiness" written all over your face, people will bombard you with their negativity and try to shoot down that positive attitude of yours.

In this article, you will find seven positive thinking tips that can help you to develop and maintain a positive outlook on life.

1. Try To Spend As Much Time As Possible With People Who Have A Positive Attitude: Let's face it - we are social creatures, and other people's attitudes affect us. So try to make use of that for yourself. **2. Exercise Can Help You To Feel Good:** Studies have shown that exercise can be as effective - and sometimes even more effective - than depression medication. When you get your heart pumping regularly, and all your cells get supplied with generous amounts of oxygen, that alone will help you to feel and think better.

3. Sleep Tight: A lot of people think that five or six hours of sleep are enough for them. But the truth is, anyone who doesn't get at least seven hours of sleep a day will suffer from some kind of sleep deprivation, which will often manifest itself in unclear thinking or mood swings. A good night's sleep, on the other hand, supplies your mind and body with all the happy hormones that can charge your positive thinking.

4. Write A Gratitude Journal: This is one of the most powerful yet most underutilized positive thinking tips of all time. Gratitude is a great source of positive thinking - yet, most people neglect it and never make proper use of it. You don't have to be grateful for big things - small things are totally fine. You could be grateful for the fact that the computer screen on which you are reading this article right now is working - that's a miracle. Not even the richest and most powerful man in the world could do that just one hundred years ago - reading words from an illuminated screen.

5. Eat Healthily: Eat lots of fresh vegetables and fruits and proteins. Eat several meals a day, enjoy your breakfast in the morning. Never feel too hungry, as it will only lead to overeating later on.

6. Be A Realistic Optimist: That means, see things for what they are - even if things don't look good right now. But believe in the potential that you have it inside yourself to make things better.

7. Use Positive Mindset Hypnosis: Your subconscious mind is a way more powerful machine that your conscious mind. You can tell yourself all the positive affirmations in the world, but that's all going to your conscious mind. With hypnosis, you can communicate directly with the most powerful part of your personality and influence it positively.

CHAPTER 10 - WHAT IS INTUITIVE EATING?

Intuitive eating is an approach to health and food that has nothing to do with diets, meal plans, discipline or willpower. It teaches you how to get in touch with your body cues like hunger, fullness, and satisfaction while learning to trust your body around food again. Here's an overview of intuitive eating including the science behind it, the ten principles of intuitive eating, and the difference between intuitive eating and mindful eating. For more info on ditching the diet and healing your relationship with food, check out the Intuitive Eating Crash Course.

What Is Intuitive Eating?

Intuitive eating is an approach that was created by two registered dietitians, Evelyn Tribole and Elyse Resch, in 1995. Intuitive eating is a non-diet approach to health and wellness that helps you tune into your body signals, break the cycle of chronic dieting and heal your relationship with food. From a nutrition professional perspective, intuitive eating is a framework that helps us keep nutrition interventions behavior-focused instead of restrictive or rule-focused.

The basics

1. Intuitive eating is an eating style that promotes a healthy attitude toward food and body image.

2. The idea is that you should eat when you're hungry and stop when you're full.
3. Though this should be an intuitive process, for many people it's not.
4. Trusting diet books and so-called experts about what, when, and how to eat can lead you away from trusting your body and its intuition.
5. To eat intuitively, you may need to relearn how to trust your body. To do that, you need to distinguish between physical and emotional hunger:

   ❖ Physical hunger. This biological urge tells you to replenish nutrients. It builds gradually and has different signals, such as a growling stomach, fatigue, or irritability. It's satisfying when you eat any food.
   ❖ Emotional hunger. This is driven by emotional needs. Sadness, loneliness, and boredom are some of the feelings that can create cravings for food, often comfort foods. Eating then causes guilt and self-hatred.

We are all born natural intuitive eaters. Babies cry, they eat, and then stop eating until they're hungry again. Kids innately balance out their food intake from week to week, eating when they're hungry and stopping once they feel full. Some days they may eat a ton of food, and other days they may eat barely anything. As we grow older and rules and restrictions are set around food, we lose our inner intuitive eater. We learn to finish everything on our plates. We learn that dessert is a reward, or can be taken away if we misbehave. We are told that certain foods are good for us and others are bad – causing us to feel good about ourselves when we eat certain foods and guilty when we eat others.

Intuitive Eating is not a diet. It's exactly the opposite. There's no counting calories or macros and no making certain foods off-limits. It's not about following a meal plan or measuring out your portions (in fact, that is all discouraged!). Instead, it's about re-learning to eat outside of the diet mentality, putting the focus on your internal cues (aka your intuition) like hunger, fullness, and satisfaction, and moving away from external cues like food rules and restrictions.

But intuitive eating is not the 'hunger-fullness diet'. Intuitive eaters give themselves unconditional permission to eat whatever they want without feeling guilty. They rely on their internal hunger and satiety signals and trust their body to tell them when what and how much to eat. They know when they want to eat veggies and also when they feel like having dessert (and don't feel guilty or have any regrets with either choice).

The Science Behind Intuitive Eating

- ❖ Higher self-esteem
- ❖ Better body image
- ❖ More satisfaction with life
- ❖ Optimism and well-being
- ❖ Proactive coping skills
- ❖ Lower body mass indexes
- ❖ Higher HDL cholesterol levels
- ❖ Lower Triglyceride levels
- ❖ Lower rates of emotional eating
- ❖ Lower rates of disordered eating

The 4 Characteristics Of Intuitive Eating Are:

- ❖ Unconditional permission to eat
- ❖ Eating for physical rather than emotional reasons
- ❖ Reliance on internal hunger and satiety cues
- ❖ Choosing foods that both make the person feel good in his or her body and taste good.

Guidelines For Intuitive Eating

- ❖ Eat when you are physically hungry.
- ❖ Eat sitting down in a calm environment.
- ❖ Eat without distractions such as radio, television, newspapers, books, intense or anxiety-provoking conversations or music.

- ❖ Eat what your body wants. (Your body, not your spoiled inner child!)
- ❖ Eat to be in full view of others.
- ❖ Eat with enjoyment, gusto, and pleasure.
- ❖ Stop when you are full.

By committing to adopt and implement these guidelines, you will find yourself firmly planted on the path to anxiety-free eating and weight loss, something I wish everyone caught on the diet treadmill could discover.

Benefits Of Intuitive Eating

Intuitive eating is not designed for weight loss. Unfortunately, there may be dietitians, coaches, and other practitioners that sell intuitive eating as a diet, which runs counter to the idea entirely.

The goal of intuitive eating is to improve your relationship with food. This includes building healthier food behaviors and not trying to manipulate the scale. Of course, that being said, almost every single person going through the process of learning to be an intuitive eater wants to lose weight otherwise, they'd already been intuitive eaters!

Intuitive eating allows your body to break the diet cycle and settle into its natural set point weight range. This may be lower, higher, or the same weight you are right now. It can help you lose weight if you find yourself eating for reasons that have little to do with how hungry or full you are, and more to do with specific feelings or personal triggers.

There don't seem to be any downsides to intuitive eating, so I'm certainly encouraging of anyone giving it a shot. When you take away some powerful triggers in your everyday life that attribute value to the food, you get a much better sense of what you feel in a given moment and why you want to eat and when.

Overall Health Benefits

Intuitive eating has been shown to have both physical and emotional health benefits.

- Improved cholesterol levels
- Lower rates of emotional and disordered eating
- Better body image
- Higher self-esteem
- Reduced stress
- Improved metabolism
- Higher levels of contentment and satisfaction

A review included 24 cross-sectional studies that examined the psychosocial effect intuitive eating had on adult women. Intuitive eating was associated with the following positive results:

- Less disordered eating
- More positive body image

❖ Greater emotional functioning

What's The Difference Between Intuitive Eating And Mindful Eating?

Before I started training in Intuitive Eating, I used the terms Mindful Eating and Intuitive Eating interchangeably. While this isn't incorrect, it's important to note the differences.

The Center for Mindful Eating defines mindful eating as "allowing yourself to become aware of the positive and nurturing opportunities that are available through food selection and preparation by respecting your inner wisdom" and "using all your senses in choosing to eat food that is both satisfying to you and nourishing to your body and becoming aware of physical hunger and satiety cues to guide your decisions to begin and end eating."

You can tell right there that Intuitive Eating encompasses the principles of mindful eating. However it goes a step further, also addressing the importance of rejecting the dieting mentality, respecting your body (regardless of your weight or shape), coping with emotional eating, and gentle movement and nutrition without judgment. Both mindful eating and Intuitive Eating can be useful tools to help you reach a place of normal eating.

Steps To Becoming An Intuitive And Mindful Eater

Diets are all about restriction. Someone hands you a meal or a diet book that lays out a specific plan of what you can eat when you can eat it, how much you should eat and how long you should follow this set of "rules" to reach your goal. The problem with this is once the diet is "over", the weight has a tendency to come back, because there is no longer a road map to follow.

You may have read or heard the terms "intuitive eating" and "mindful eating". These terms are often used interchangeably and while they are related, they are also different. Both, however, are key to finally getting off the diet roller coaster.

Intuitive eating is eating based on your physiological hunger and satiety signals and not based on situations and emotions. Mindful eating is about paying attention to the act of eating, without judgment. It is an important step on your journey to becoming an intuitive eater. When you eat mindfully, you are more aware of your eating habits, the sensations you experience when you eat, the taste, texture, and aroma of the food, and the thoughts and emotions that you have about food. It is more about how you eat than what you eat.

Many of the issues that dieters face come from a lack of tuning into certain feelings and cues while eating. Then they punish themselves for overeating and move on to another diet with a new set of restrictions.

There are 3 crucial steps that you need to take to become an intuitive eater. First, you need to develop a non-diet mindset; second, you need caring support and third, you need to honor your body. No form of dieting is going to work for you to lose the weight and keep it off. These three steps are crucial to be freed of dieting forever.

1. **Step One:** Shifting into a non-diet mindset is all about rejecting the diet mentality. You likely have a list of "good" and "bad", or "legal" or "Illegal" foods that you can or cannot eat. This sets you up for feelings of deprivation and eventual overheating on those foods you have deprived yourself of. Throwing out those lists and the diets you have in your home will set your commitment to a diet-free way of life.

2. **Step Two:** Building a strong support network is important to help cheer you along. Equally important, if not more important, is the aspect of self-care. You must take care of your basic needs if you expect to be able to tune into your inner signals. Take time for yourself, get enough sleep, and schedule playtime into your busy day.

3. **Step Three:** Honoring your body by tuning into your thoughts, feelings, and signals. This means to listen for your

hunger signals and your fullness signals and let those signals guide your eating at every meal.

The process of learning to become an intuitive and mindful eater is a journey. It is about taking steps towards becoming someone you love inside and out. It will end your search for the next diet miracle because it is through intuitive and mindful eating that you will find your destination: a body you love and that you can maintain forever without dieting.

8 Tips For Intuitive Eating

Interested in giving intuitive eating a try? Here are eight things to keep in mind.

- ❖ The principles (and caveats) below provide a basic road map for increasing your food awareness and satisfaction. Intuitive eaters eat when hungry and to satisfy their cravings but they stay ever mindful of their physiology, experience, and state of mind.

- ❖ Learn to recognize mild sensations of hunger that emerge even while you are busy doing something else, and feed them before you become ravenous or become tempted to make unhealthy eating choices.

- ❖ Give yourself permission to eat whenever you feel hungry, and let go of internal feelings of guilt or rigid rules that say you can't eat more than a certain number of calories a day or enjoy a slice of cake.

- ❖ Derive pleasure and satisfaction from the eating experience moment by moment, without distraction, and savor your food. Notice when and how your hunger abates. While you are eating, do not watch television, work at the computer or think about your plans for the rest of the day. Instead, look at your food, observing color, shape, taste, smell, texture, and quality. Observe your sensations and reactions.

- ❖ After a meal is done, take some time to focus on your inner feelings sluggish or energized, anxious or calm? Decide whether the meal and its contents are worth eating again.

- ❖ Don't eat to alleviate anxiety, boredom or depression. If you find yourself overeating to treat a mood or emotion instead of to satisfy physiological hunger, search for the emotional root of the problem and then soothe or stimulate yourself through yoga, a long walk, or talk with a friend.

- ❖ Exercise and move for enjoyment not expressly for weight loss or calorie burning.

- ❖ Notice how you feel when you choose healthy, high-quality food. Take stock of your physical, mental, and emotional responses.

Keep caveats in mind: Many integrative health experts point out that the foods we most crave are sometimes those to which we are allergic or intolerant. If you suffer from this sort of food "addiction," be aware that feeding it may make your cravings worse

5 Intuitive Eating Mistakes You Don't Want To Make

Something I've been noticing is that there's confusion around intuitive eating and how it can help with transforming our relationship with food.

The whole premise of intuitive or mindful eating, as I shared in this post and this post, is that when we eat intuitively, we listen to our unique body's hunger and fullness signals, and honor our body by choosing high quality, whole foods that will nourish us, and to take the time to eat and enjoy food using all our senses.

When we take the time to tune into our body and to truly savor the food we eat, and when used in combination with my blueprint for having more fun and pleasure in our lives, then it's much easier to stop the dieting mindset, put an end to emotional eating and to overcome overeating and binge eating. However, there are some traps that I see people getting into when they embark on the intuitive eating journey which can sabotage their efforts to move into a healthier lifestyle.

Mistake 1 Using Intuitive Eating As An Excuse To Eat Whatever And Whenever You Want

Yes, with intuitive eating you are encouraged to let go of control and restriction and to allow yourself to eat what you like. However, it's also about treating your body with respect and listening and feeling into your body and what it truly needs and wants.

When you're eating intuitively, it's unlikely you will desire junk food all of the time, and if you're honoring your hunger and fullness cues then it's unlikely you will want to eat anything and everything. When you start listening to your body, you will likely notice that if you eat crappy food, you just feel lethargic, bloated and blah; but if you eat well, then you feel energized, satisfied and nourished. There is no doubt that it takes practice to learn how your body works, but when you do heal your relationship with your body by eating intuitively then it becomes second nature and you will be able to ditch the diet books for good.

Mistake 2 Holding Onto The Diet Mentality

Another key element of intuitive eating is that this is NOT another diet. The reason that the majority of people end up over-eating, and gaining weight is that they have yo-yo dieted all their lives. For most, the years of diet obsession and focusing on ways to manipulate body size have only caused a lack of return- in money, time, and energy.

Despite this, the mental conditioning from years of dieting can make it difficult to try an approach like this that requires you to trust your body, find your natural body size and focus on healthy behaviors rather than the numbers on a scale. It can be downright terrifying to let go of the diet thinking, but being open to the intuitive eating approach and giving it a proper go is what will eventually lead to body and food freedom.

Mistake 3 Using Intuitive Eating As A Tool To Lose Weight

With intuitive eating, the end goal is not weight loss. The idea is that intuitive eating will give your body a chance to reach its set-point weight range- and this can only happen when eating and exercise have been normal for several months. Some people do gain weight when they first start intuitive eating, while others will lose weight. But this shouldn't be the focus- healthy behaviors are what is important.

Once you're living healthily, then the body will reach its set point weight naturally and this is what will bring the mind and body transformation that will allow you to also live without obsessing about the numbers on the scale all of the time. Finding a way to have peace with your body size and by accepting that healthy behavior are more important than weight are the key.

Mistake 4 Continuing To Restrict Or Control Your Food

When people start using their willpower and self-control to eat mindfully perfectly, it is just an extension of the "diet mentality" that we are all so used to. Mindful eating is about letting go of willpower and self-control, and simply tuning into the body's needs in the present moment. When eating intuitively, it's time to release the mind of all the rules and tools such as weighing food grams, measuring portion sizes and counting calories. These tools are not needed when we are in tune with our body and how it feels and what it craves.

Healthy habits that can be maintained, rely on being created based on your body's internal wisdom, not by external tools which tell you what to do all the time. It's useful to remember that intuitive eating is a moment-to-moment daily practice of mindfulness which allows you to be free from the reactive, habitual patterns of being on a diet.

Mistake 5 Judging Your Success And Failure

Following intuitive eating requires continual practice- it is lifelong learning and not a test that you can fail or succeed at it. Thinking this way will only keep you in self-judgment and the diet mentality- which is likely how you got to the place of needing to overcome cravings and put an end to over-eating in the first place. With intuitive eating, there is no such thing as perfection, and there is no need to try and strive to eat 100% intuitively all the time to be perfect.

Instead, when you eat, be aware of your thoughts, emotions, and feelings in the present moment without judgment. Let go of perfection and the idea that you must eat mindfully 100% of the time or that you can't eat a certain type of food. This is not another diet in another guise- it's a whole new paradigm of thinking and living.

Intuitive Eating Mistakes You Don't Want To Make

Instead of judging yourself, be curious and notice your thoughts. Rather than judging your progress by looking at your weight or level of restriction, start focussing on indicators such as how well you listened to your hunger and fullness cues, whether you honored your cravings, and also by being aware of your negative thoughts and disordered behaviors and patterns learned from your past if they creep in.

Avoiding these five mistakes is important for being successful with intuitive eating. Remember that it's a moment-by-moment daily practice, and the benefits that it will bring to your life will make any challenges 100% worth it. This approach will always be better than other diet methods you have unsuccessfully tried in the past and will help you to live a life where you are no longer controlled by food or obsessed with your weight, and allow you to live your life fully and happily.

Principles Of Intuitive Eating

1. Reject The Diet Mentality

Throw out the diet books and magazine articles that offer you the false hope of losing weight quickly, easily, and permanently. Get angry at diet culture that promotes weight loss and the lies that have led you to feel as if you were a failure every time a new diet stopped working and you gained back all of the weight. If you allow even one small hope to linger that a new and better diet or food plan might be lurking around the corner, it will prevent you from being free to rediscover Intuitive Eating.

2. Honor Your Hunger

Keep your body biologically fed with adequate energy and carbohydrates. Otherwise, you can trigger a primal drive to overeat. Once you reach the moment of excessive hunger, all intentions of moderate, conscious eating are fleeting and irrelevant. Learning to honor this first biological signal sets the stage for rebuilding trust in yourself and food.

3. Make Peace With Food

Call a truce; stop the food fight! Give yourself unconditional permission to eat. If you tell yourself that you can't or shouldn't have a particular food, it can lead to intense feelings of deprivation that build into uncontrollable cravings and, often, bingeing. When you finally "give in" to your forbidden foods, eating will be experienced with such intensity it usually results in Last Supper overeating and overwhelming guilt.

4. Challenge The Food Police

Scream a loud no to thoughts in your head that declare you're "good" for eating minimal calories or "bad" because you ate a piece of chocolate cake. The food police monitor the unreasonable rules that diet culture has created. The police station is housed deep in your psyche, and its loud speaker shouts negative barbs, hopeless phrases, and guilt-provoking indictments. Chasing the Food Police away is a critical step in returning to Intuitive Eating.

5. Discover The Satisfaction Factor

The Japanese have the wisdom to keep pleasure as one of their goals of healthy living. In our compulsion to comply with diet culture, we often overlook one of the most basic gifts of existence—the pleasure and satisfaction that can be found in the eating experience. When you eat what you want, in an environment that is inviting, the pleasure you derive will be a powerful force in helping you feel satisfied and content. By providing this experience for yourself, you will find that it takes just the right amount of food for you to decide you've had "enough."

6. Feel Your Fullness

To honor your fullness, you need to trust that you will give yourself the foods that you desire. Listen to the body signals that tell you that you are no longer hungry. Observe the signs that show that you're comfortably full. Pause in the middle of eating and ask yourself how the food tastes, and what your current hunger level is.

7. Cope With Your Emotions With Kindness

First, recognize that food restriction, both physically and mentally, can, in and of itself, trigger loss of control, which can feel like emotional eating. Find kind ways to comfort, nurture, distract, and resolve your issues. Anxiety, loneliness, boredom, and anger are emotions we all experience throughout life. Each has its trigger, and each has its appeasement. Food won't fix any of these feelings. It may comfort for the short term, distract from the pain, or even numb you. But the food won't solve the problem. If anything, eating for an emotional hunger may only make you feel worse in the long run. You'll ultimately have to deal with the source of the emotion.

8. Respect Your Body

Accept your genetic blueprint. Just as a person with a shoe size of eight would not expect to realistically squeeze into a size six, it is equally futile (and uncomfortable) to have a similar expectation about body size. But mostly, respect your body so you can feel better about who you are. It's hard to reject the diet mentality if you are unrealistic and overly critical of your body size or shape. All bodies deserve dignity.

9. Movement Feel The Difference

Forget militant exercise. Just get active and feel the difference. Shift your focus to how it feels to move your body, rather than the calorie-burning effect of exercise. If you focus on how you feel from working out, such as energized, it can make the difference between rolling out of bed for a brisk morning walk or hitting the snooze alarm.

10. Honor Your Health-Gentle Nutrition

Make food choices that honor your health and taste buds while making you feel good. Remember that you don't have to eat perfectly to be healthy. You will not suddenly get a nutrient deficiency or become unhealthy, from one snack, one meal, or one day of eating. It's what you eat consistently over time that matters. Progress, not perfection, is what counts.

Powerful Weight Loss Tip

Stop dieting and start eating consciously in a way that makes your body feel well. Eating with intuition is different for every person, but the general aspect of listening to your body remains constant. Time and again, research has proven that dieting for weight loss is not sustainable. Besides, it causes more harm than good to your body and mind. Dieting increases the risk of eating disorders, binge eating, weight cycling, and weight stigma.

In my practice, I find that more people can achieve their personal best weight with intuitive eating than with traditional dieting. I suggest you give it a try. Intuitive Eating is based on interoceptive awareness or the ability to perceive physical sensations inside your body. This means, to be able to eat intuitively, you need to connect with your body and listen to your body's "messages."

In contrast, focusing on weight loss is based on external rules. It dulls your interoceptive sense and leads to body-doubt. It makes you think that something is wrong with you just because you're not losing weight as you expected. Thus, you're likely to think that intuitive eating "doesn't work." While it's true that some people lose weight when they eat intuitively, weight loss is more of a side effect rather than the focal point of intuitive eating. Some people who eat intuitively don't lose weight, and that's okay.

Intuitive eating is weight neutral and is aligned with the Health At Every Size approach. These 3 steps will guide you in getting started.

1. Eat When You Are Hungry

Watch for your body's hunger cues as your signal that it is time to eat. Eat enough to feel satisfied and comfortably full, not stuffed. For most people, this means eating every 3-4 hours or so. Balanced meals that include whole grains, protein foods, vegetables, fruits, dairy products, and healthy fats promote satisfaction and satiety.

2. Eat What You Want

If you don't, you'll likely feel deprived and find yourself overeating. Restricting yourself from certain foods may also keep you on the hunt for food whether you're hungry or not. If you notice that what you want is always the richer choice, you may still be caught up in feeling deprived of years of dieting. Try compromising by using richer foods in smaller quantities. For example, use real butter to spread on a small piece of your favorite crusty bread.

3. Eat Until You've Had Enough

If you are used to eating until you're uncomfortably full, you may need to work on redefining your definition of how much is enough. You may have normalized feeling stuffed. Consistently eating this way is not good for your health and it probably means that you are not listening to your body's signal of fullness. Occasional overeating is normal; it's the habit that you want to avoid.

CHAPTER 11 - BODY RESPECT

What Does It Mean To Have Respect For Your Body?

Body respect means feeding your body and knowing (deeply) that your body deserves to be fed. It means dressing your body in comfortable clothes and not squeezing her into fabric she doesn't fit in. It means touching your body with affection and moving your body in comfortable and life-affirming ways

The language around bodies and health can be confusing and oftentimes misleading. When Alissa and I begin work with clients to heal their body image, we often hear: "It seems like I'm just supposed to wake up one day and suddenly love everything about my body that's never going to happen!" We're grateful for such awesome clients who open up and share these thoughts with us because – yes, it is unrealistic!

Diet culture messages imply or directly say that to be healthy, to be happy and to be successful you must be thin. And while hashtags like #bodylove and #bodypositive started as a way to promote positive body image messages, at this point it often feels like these hashtags have been taken over by thin women with socially acceptable body types. This can make the idea of loving your body even more daunting.

This is why we like to shift from thinking about loving your body to instead working on moving towards feeling neutral about your body and respecting your body. Can you move from body dissatisfaction to body neutrality? Can you spend less time thinking about and worrying about your body, even if you don't love it looks? And can you respect your body no matter how you feel about it?

Body Love vs Body Respect

Newsflash: you don't have to love everything about your body and it's unrealistic to think we will love every single thing about our bodies. This is where body respect comes in: it is really difficult to take good care of something that you don't respect. So rather than a goal of loving your body, aiming for body respect is more realistic and ultimately more important when it comes to taking care of yourself.

Even on the days when you may not feel your body 'looks' up to your standards, it's still doing so many things to keep you alive and participating in your life. Think about all the amazing things our bodies do for us: it allows us to hug our loved ones, birth babies, participate in social activities, convert food into energy, and even just get out of bed in the morning.

These are all things that, regardless of how you feel about your body image today, your body is still doing for you or helping you do. So what does body respect look like? Here are some examples:

- ❖ Honoring your hunger signals, eating something every time your body tells you that it's hungry.
- ❖ Dressing in clothes that fit and feel comfortable.
- ❖ Talking to yourself with compassion and kindness
- ❖ Moving your body in a way that feels good to you

Bodies are meant to look and be different. And regardless of what they look like on the outside, they're doing a lot for you on the inside. Try to take some time to think about the following questions:

- ❖ How would you respect your body more if it looked differently?
- ❖ How does waiting until you look a certain way to give yourself respect align with your values?
- ❖ What would it be like to take care of your body and show it respect now, instead of waiting until you reach a certain goal?
- ❖ What would it be like to eat and move in a way that felt good instead of in the hopes of changing your body?
- ❖ What would it feel like to spend less time preoccupied with how your body looks or you wished it looked?

6 Ways To Practice Body Respect

1. Diversify Your Social Media Feed: We say this all the time over here, but diversifying the images you see and the messages you get about bodies, health, food, and beauty is a huge step towards feeling better in your body. Here are some of the favorite Instagram accounts that feature a variety of diverse body sizes, shapes, ages, genders, abilities, and colors.

2. Buy Comfortable Clothes: If your clothes (this includes underwear and bras) are tight or don't fit well, it will be a constant daily reminder. Don't wait until you are at a certain size to buy new clothes – dress the body that you have now. Treat your body with respect by buying yourself clothes that fit you, clothes that you like, and clothes that you feel comfortable in.

3. Practice Self-Care: Do nice things for your body. Think about ways that you can take care of your body, both physically and mentally. This could be meditation, deep breathing, movement, running a bubble bath, watching a favorite tv show, taking a walk with a friend, using some luxurious body lotion, or reading a good book. Check out this blog post on Building a Self-Care Toolbox for more ideas.

4. Stop Body Checking And Comparing Yourself To Others: Remind yourself that you don't know anyone else's story. They may have the "perfect" body, but you don't know what's going on inside of them. We all look different and bodies come in all shapes and sizes. Body diversity exists naturally and it is a beautiful thing. Try to catch yourself when you find yourself comparing yourself to others and put the focus back on yourself.

5. Don't Tear Apart Your Body: When you're feeling down about yourself or your body, work on not spiraling into a negative script of things you're unhappy with or wish to change. Instead, think about how you'd talk to and support a friend who was feeling the same way. What would you say to them? You'd likely show them much more compassion than you do yourself. Try to then show that same compassion to yourself and stop the negative self-talk in its tracks.

6. Focus On What Your Body Does For You: What are some compliments you can give yourself that have nothing to do with what you look like? Make a list of at least 15 things that you like about yourself. If this is difficult, think about the things you love and appreciate about your friends and loved ones. When you do give compliments to others, try to do so in a way that has nothing to do with their looks or their body. Some ideas: "Your smile lights up the room!"; "You're a great listener"; "Thank you for always showing up and making me feel heard"; "You are so fun to be around"; or "I love the way you think."

Ways To Respect Your Body

Have you ever looked in the mirror and disparaged all the parts of you that you wish you could change? I think it's safe to say we've all been there. But in the same way that wearing a shoe that's too small won't magically shrink your foot, shaming your body is not going to make it look any different or make you feel better about who you are.

Here Are 10 Ways You Can Start Being Kind To Your Body And Give It The Respect It Deserves:

1. **Compliment Yourself:** Appreciate and remind yourself of the parts of your body that you like the best.

2. **Talkback To Negative Thoughts:** Pay attention to how often you find yourself bashing your body (or the bodies of others) and don't let those thoughts go unchecked. Work to actively replace those comments with kind statements.

3. **Stop Weighing Yourself:** No number will ever truly be good enough so this practice is unlikely to help you feel happier about your body.

4. Wear clothing that is comfortable, flattering, and fits you without being too tight or hides your body in too baggy of clothing regardless of the size.

5. **Stop Comparing Yourself To Others:** No one body is the "right" kind of body. Therefore, how can your body be "wrong?"

6. **Avoid Dieting To "Slim Down" Before A Big Event:** Your capability of having a great time and making lasting memories is not contingent on losing weight.

7. **Allow Your Body To Experience A Soothing Touch:** Take a bubble bath, get a massage and hug people you feel comfortable hugging. Everybody craves and deserves a soothing touch.

8. **Honor Your Hunger:** When you recognize your physical hunger signals, make the time to eat. Ignoring that communication from your body will cause yourself to be over-hungry and then it's difficult to determine what you want to eat and when you have had enough.

9. **Honor your fullness:** Slow down your pace at meals to allow your body to enjoy the experience of eating. Pause in the middle of your meal to check in with your level of fullness and ask yourself how the food tastes. Then, when you observe the signs that you are comfortably full, give your body the gift of stopping before you are uncomfortably full.

10. Be Realistic About Your Genetic Makeup And Realize That All Bodies Are Different: When you are practicing self-care, honoring your hunger and fullness signals and moving in ways that feel good your body will likely balance out at its natural weight. Note that I did not say "ideal weight." Ideal weight is a fictional concept because all bodies are different and not one is ideal.

Forgive Yourself For Your Mistakes

Letting go of the past can be difficult, but to respect who you are now, you must let go of who you were then. Do whatever you can to forgive yourself for mistakes you've made. We've all made them it's part of life but those who respect themselves know how to let those mistakes go. You can never go back; you can only take what's happened and move positively forward.

Forgive Those Who Have Hurt You

Forgiveness can be tough sometimes, especially if you've been hurt badly. But caring around that hurt and anger only makes it more difficult to cultivate love within yourself. Let go of the pain others have caused and you'll open up space in your heart in mind for more positive emotions and experiences. No matter what wrong has been committed against you, forgiving is always better than clinging to the pain.

Surround Yourself With Positive People

Respecting yourself means keeping company with those who respect you and themselves. Negative people (even those who are not negative directly to you) are draining and they spark negative thought patterns within you. You've heard the old saying: you are a combination of the people you spend the most time with. Respect yourself enough to make sure those people are positive influences.

Work On Building Up Confidence

The more you believe in yourself, the easier it will be to treat yourself with love and respect. Confidence isn't always easy to come by, however, so you've gotta work for it. Do things that you're good at. Accept compliments and make note of when others are proud of you. The more you do things that build up your confidence (and avoid those that tear it down), the more confident you'll feel. And the more confident you are, the less likely you are to settle.

Be Honest With Yourself (And Others)

Honesty is the ultimate sign of respect. When you're honest with yourself, you'll see what's good for you and what's not. You'll be less likely to compromise on what matters most to you. Being honest with yourself is pretty hard to pay attention to how you feel and what you think. And practice the art of being honest with others. Even when it's hard, the truth is always the way to go.

Take Good Care Of Your Body

Making yourself feel good physically is one of the ultimate ways to respect yourself. Treat your body as you would the body of someone you love dearly. Healthy food, exercise, low stress. Respecting your body is an essential aspect of self-respect. The more kindness you show yourself physically, the more internal love you'll feel. Your body is the vessel transporting you around this world and it's up to you to respect it.

Exercise And Inspire Your Mind

Just as you need to respect your body, you also need to respect your mind. Challenge yourself with new experiences and information. Step out of the thinking you're comfortable with and try to find new perspectives. Find resources for information and inspiration books, websites, people and soak up all you can. The more you know, the more you can grow. And all that growth will empower you, making it much easier to respect yourself.

Speak Positively About Yourself

The way you speak about yourself says a lot about how much respect you have for who you are. Try always to speak about yourself positively and try never to put yourself down with negativity. If this is a struggle for you, check out Using Positive Words to Promote Self-Love, which will give you inspiration for speaking positively about yourself. (Plus there's a free download with lots and lots of words!)

Don't Compare Yourself To Others

Theodore Roosevelt rightly said, "Comparison is the thief of joy." The more you compare your life to someone else's, the more difficult it becomes to cultivate self-respect. It's hard not to compare, but remind yourself that, no matter how well you know someone, you don't even know everything about his or her life. No life is perfect and an essential way to respect yourself is to focus on what you have, not on what you lack.

What Is Body Language?

Body Language is the unspoken, nonverbal communication that goes on in every Face-to-Face encounter with another human being. It tells you their true feelings towards you and how well your words are being received. Between 50-100% of our message is communicated through our Body Language. A simple roll of the eyes or hand gesture may be all it takes to convey 100% of what we mean, no words, no tone, in fact only 7-10% is attributable to the actual words we use.

Your ability to read and understand another person's Body Language can mean the difference between making a great impression or a very bad one! It doesn't matter how clever or knowledgeable you are in your field, if you can't get your point across effectively or decode other people you work with then you're at a disadvantage to those that do.

Here Are Ten Practical Tips On Using Body Language To Improve Your Life.

1.Eye Contact: Eye contact is one of the most important aspects of dealing with others, especially people we have just met. Maintaining good eye contact shows respect and interest in what they have to say. In the UK we tend to keep eye contact around 60-70% of the time giving a feeling of comfort and genuine warmth in your company. Any more eye contact than this and you can be too intense, any less and you give off a signal that you are lacking interest in them or their conversation.

2.Posture: Posture is the next thing to master, get your posture right and you will automatically start feeling better, as it makes you feel good almost instantly. Next time you notice you are feeling a bit down, take a look at how you are standing or sitting. Chances are you will be slouched over with your shoulders drooping down and inward. This collapses the chest and inhibits good breathing, which in turn can help make you feel nervous or uncomfortable.

3.Head Position: When you want to feel confident and self-assured keep your head level both horizontally and vertically. You can also use this straight head position when you want to be authoritative and have what you are saying to be taken seriously. Conversely, when you want to be friendly and in the listening, receptive mode, tilt your head just a little to one side or other.

4.Arms: In general terms the more outgoing you are as a person, the more you tend to use your arms with big movements. The quieter you are the less you move your arms away from your body. So, try to strike a natural balance. When you want to come across in the best possible light, crossing the arms is a no, no in front of others. If someone says something that gets your goat, then, by all means, show your disapproval by crossing them!

5.Legs: Legs are the furthest point away from the brain; consequently, they are the hardest bits of our bodies to consciously control. They tend to move around a lot more than normal when we are nervous, stressed or being deceptive. Be careful too in the way you cross your legs. If you bring your leg up to rest on the knee of the other this is known as the 'Figure Four' and is generally perceived as the most defensive leg cross.

6. Angle Of Body: The angle of the body concerning others indicates our attitudes and feelings towards them. We angle toward people we find attractive, friendly and interesting and angle ourselves away from those we do not, it is that simple!

7. Hand Gestures: Basic rules, Palms slightly up and outward is open and friendly. Palm down generally seen as dominant and possibly aggressive. This palm up, palm down is very important when it comes to handshaking and where appropriate I suggest you always offer a handshake upright and vertical and equal grip, which should convey equality.

8. Distance: Stand too close and you will be marked as 'Pushy' or 'In your face'. Stand or sit too far away and you will be 'Keeping your distance' or 'Standoffish'. Neither situation is what we want, so observe in a group situation how close all the other people are to each other. Also, notice if you move closer to someone and they back away, you are probably just a tiny bit too much in their personal space, their comfort zone. 'You have overstepped the mark' and should pull back a little.

9. Ears: Ears, yes your ears you have got two ears and only one mouth, so try to use them in that order. If you listen twice as much as you talk you come across as a good communicator who knows how to strike a balanced conversation.

10. Mouth: We purse our lips and sometimes twist them to the side when we are thinking. On another occasion, we might use this movement to hold back an angry comment we do not wish to reveal. Nevertheless, it will probably be spotted by other people and although they may not know the comment, they will get a feeling you were not too pleased.

Having respect for other people is difficult if you have no respect for yourself. The idea of self-respect is very closely related to self-confidence, but respect is more about what you do whereas confidence is about how you feel. The two go hand-in-hand. To respect your body means treating your body with the same care you would give any other valuable and irreplaceable object. Learning to respect your body is vital because when you respect your body, you are in partnership with it. You become grounded in your physical body and able to take benefit from all parts of your body.

Yes, it is indeed that respect carries reciprocal energy. Your body will honor you when you honor it. On the contrary, if you abuse or ignore it, it will break down in various ways until you learn the lesson of respect. The following are 20 ways to respect your body:

1. Your body is an amazing creation of God, so start to respect it.

2. Make the lists of all things your body. Read and add them continuously.

3. Realize what your body can do every day. Remember that your body is a living instrument, not just a decoration.

4. Make the lists of people you admire: people who inspire you and give positive things into your life, society, and world. Pay attention to your physical appearance, so it will look important to support your achievement.

5. Walk by raising your head, full of self-confidence.

6. Do not let your weight or posture avoid you to enjoy the activities you like.

7. Wear comfortable clothes that you like.

8. Count the blessings you have accepted and do not count bad lucks you have experienced.

9. Think about other things you can reach with the time and energy you have spent to worry about body and appearance.

10. Be a friend and supporter, not an enemy to your own body.

11. Think that your skin regenerates every month, your stomach regenerates every five days, your liver regenerates

every six weeks, and your bone regenerates every three months.

12. If you get up every morning, do not forget to thank your fresh body.

13. When you want to sleep every night, do not forget to say to your body how valuable your body is in helping you do duties every day.

14. Find out the exercise method you enjoy and do regularly, but do not exercise to lower your weight or abuse your body. Do exercise for your health and body strength because it can make you pleasant.

15. Remember when you feel pleased with your body and say to yourself that you can feel it anymore, even when you have been old.

16. Make 10 lists of positive things about yourself without mentioning physical appearance.

17. Make a note and stick it out in the mirror that you look interesting both inside and outside.

18. Find the beautiful things of the world and yourself.

19. Start to say to yourself that life is too short to spent time to hate your own body.

20. Eat when you are hungry and take a rest when you feel tired. Additionally, find friends that can remind you about your beauty both inside and outside.

CHAPTER 12 - MEAL PLANNING

How To Meal Plan

If you're not familiar with meal plans for weight loss, they are a proven system of recipes and meals to eat throughout the week. Those who can stick to them see their figures shrink, and their body starts to look great. They can help you reduce the amount of work it takes to lose weight by the meals you eat, especially if you've never really come up with a meal plan of your own.

Understanding The Process

There are several different types of these plans available. A great example of this is the person who wants to cut the carbs from their diet. It's not something we recommend, but we know plenty of people who take this route. The entire plan revolves around you eating certain foods that take the place of carbohydrates. However, this works for the person who wants to watch their calorie intake, who wants to calorie shift, or any other method out there.

What Plans Are Available?

Again, this comes down to what type of diet you want for your body. If you want to lose weight, but the pack on muscle then your meals will consist of proteins. The truth is it doesn't matter what you need, because there are options for quick weight loss for everyone. The only thing you have to figure out is whether or not this approach fits in your budget, or if you can be disciplined enough to stick with it.

It's Expensive Right?

Well, it depends on how you look at it. We understand you can hit the fast-food drive-thrus and order a couple of sandwiches off the dollar menu, but taking a healthier approach with your food can alleviate those other issues down the road. Weight gain is one of them, but things such as heart disease, diabetes, and various other issues can all surface because of the plans you it. Medical bills surrounding these problems are extremely expensive.

Plus, if you go to the grocery and purchase everything needed it's going to be cheaper. The only difference is you're paying for everything upfront instead of day by day. We strongly consider looking over your budget, because in most cases you can save tons of money by eliminating fast food and other restaurants.

A meal plan diet is a healthy choice for long term weight loss. There are hundreds of diet plans to choose from. Some have weathered the test of time and others are just popping onto the horizon. If you're like most people you have gone from plan to plan to look for the right one to fit you. The plan itself can be the biggest determinant of whether you lose weight or not. Regardless of what it promises, if it is poorly put together, you won't lose weight. Run the other way when you see a diet plan that promises to lose weight quickly and easily. Weight loss is hard work; it takes discipline and determination. It is much harder to lose weight than it was to put it on. The most effective diet plan is one that allows you to lose weight and keep it off.

A Meal Plan Diet Has Many Advantages:

1. It Helps You To Eat Healthily: When planning meals, you pick foods from each of the required food groups to make up each meal. When you eat healthily, your body works better and learns how to burn fat more efficiently. When your metabolism increases, you burn more calories.

2. It Gives You Flexibility: You can vary the types of food you eat as long as you stay within the boundaries of the meal plan diet. Foods that on some diet plans might be called cheating, you can eat, because by incorporating some of these 'wants' into your meal plan, it just becomes part of the meal. You can't have pizza every meal but you can make the plan a lot easier to stick with by including some of your favorite foods in moderation.

3. It Helps With Portion Control: Many times we know how many calories we want to eat for the day but we struggle to get the right mix of nutrients. How many calories from fat, carbohydrates or fiber do we need? A well-designed meal plan diet will plan all that out for you.

4. Saves Money And Time: By planning your meals ahead of time, you can save money at the grocery store by not buying food on impulse. You make your list and stick to it. Planning your meals also keeps you from eating fast food, even if you pick something off the healthy menu.

Most meal plan diets recommend that you eat several small meals throughout the day. This keeps your body's metabolism running at a higher rate, thereby burning calories more efficiently. 5 meals made up of about 300 calories each gives most people the needed calories to stay healthy and feel full and just a few enough to be able to lose weight.

Delicious Meal Plans For Weight Loss

Eating healthy doesn't have to be hard nor does it have to be complicated trying to select meal plans for weight loss. In order to trigger your body to transition into fat-burning mode, you have to feed it multiple moderate meals per day. The best diet plan for losing weight is roughly 5 small healthy meals per day all equal in nutritional value. By constantly feeding your body small meals throughout the day you will accomplish 2 vital keys to burning fat. Firstly, you signal your metabolism to burn fuel at a faster rate because it realizes that you are eating more frequently, as opposed to hoarding on to your fat. After all, you are eating only 3 meals or less per day. Secondly, by eating more frequently you will feel fuller though out the day and curb your cravings.

The ideal meal plans for weight loss are completely customizable & interchangeable. These 10 sample meal plans for weight loss are broken up into breakfast, lunch, and dinner with two snacks in between. As long as you don't replace a breakfast meal for a lunch or dinner meal & keep your serving portions the same you should have no problems switching out meals of your preference. The best way is to have these meals prepared in advance for the week that way you will not have to worry about prep time.

Breakfast

- ❖ 3oz of Lamb or Pork sausage, Mushrooms, and spinach & a teaspoon of coconut oil Or 2 Eggs (poached or scrambled)with Spinach, Canadian Bacon, Sprouted grain bread or apple
- ❖ Snack
- ❖ 1oz of Almonds or walnuts along with a pear Or Sliced celery and carrots

Lunch

- ❖ 4 oz of grilled or baked chicken or turkey (dark meat) with carrot Sticks of Brown Rice alongside Green Salad w/apple cider vinegar and olive oil Or 3 oz of grilled shrimp with avocado & cooked Lentils
- ❖ Snack
- ❖ Half oz of Macadamia Nut butter along with Celery sticks and Carrot Sticks Or Small Green apple & 2 hard-boiled eggs

Dinner

5 oz beef steak 1 cup of steamed carrots and cauliflower & 2 teaspoons of natural butter Or 4 oz of chicken thighs or legs. Spinach (sautéed in coconut oil), ½ cup of Couscous alongside Cucumber and tomato salad with Apple Cider vinegar and olive oil.

So as you can see, it is insanely easy to eat healthily and lose weight. These sample meal plans for weight loss can be used as the foundation of your diet plan. This should give you a good idea of how a well-balanced and healthy eating regimen should consist of. By adhering to this plan you will undoubtedly lose weight and provide your body with outstanding sources of nutrition with every meal. Take this outline and use it for the next 2 weeks. Allow your body to adjust to it and make any slight modification that you need to. From there you will have a core understanding of how to assemble an intelligent diet plan. The key thing to remember is to keep your serving portions moderate and to eat 5 times a day. With these 10 meal plans for weight loss, you now have a concrete plan as to what you can eat. Take this plan and use it to achieve your weight loss success.

Top Tips To Meal Planning For Weight Loss

A well-planned diet is truly essential to weight loss. This is the reason behind dieters being encouraged to pay special attention to what they eat. And if you are aiming for a sexier and leaner you, then efforts should be made to achieve your goal of losing weight. Meal planning for weight loss is indeed critical, which is why you need to be watchful and mindful about it. With this said, the following are some top tips you can follow to help you reach your ultimate objective and that is to lose the extra pounds.

Know The Essentials

Calories are that bad especially if you can burn them upon intake. They are packets of energy that are essential for cellular and multi-cellular functions. So, you should not rush into eliminating calories from your diet altogether. Instead, you have to stick to your recommended intake per day. Moreover, you should make an effort to familiarize yourself with other food groups that will help your cause. With knowledge of these things, you become more able to plan your meals much more carefully. In which case, you can prepare your meals instead of relying on diet meal delivery services.

Keep A Food Diary

It will help you out if can make a list of your diet for about a week. If you are not exactly sure how to go about this meal planning for weight loss, you can consult diet menu plans to get great ideas. From there on, you can then come up with a more creative plan for your diet.

Be Flexible In Creating The Meal Plan

It is certainly good to stick with a stringent diet but there are instances when you may have instant cravings. This is why you need to create a flexible diet plan to give way to these changes in your mood and appetite. It is then suggested that you come up with a general meal plan that can cover a variety of options for breakfasts, lunches as well as dinners.

Utilize Carb-Trimming And Timing

Carb trimming is especially difficult for individuals who have been so used to having a dose of carbohydrates in their diet. If you are struggling in this matter, what you want to do is to utilize carb-timing instead. You do not necessarily have to avoid carbohydrates intake altogether. Most individuals have already proven the advantage of such a timing strategy. For instance, you can enjoy a healthy dose of carbohydrates in your breakfast or lunch. However, you must take it away from your night meals. This way, you can still strike a balance in your diet.

Get A Healthy Dose Of Vegetables

Vegetables will do you good which is why you need to make it the center of your diet. It does not mean however that you have to forget all about the tasteful ingredients including cream and bacon. However, you should practice discipline in using them.

You only need them in small amounts. Such is enough to add the kind of flavor you are craving for in your meal. In this way, you can enjoy a healthy yet still satisfying meal. And these tips will help you with effective meal planning for weight loss.

What Is A Healthy Diet Meal Plan?

Normally people think that health is a state of a living being where there is no disease and it is really difficult to describe that what health is but for sure health can be maintained with the help of good habits and a healthy diet meal plan. Adopting healthy eating habits is the most significant part to maintain good health. Healthy meal plans for weight loss is only one of your options in losing extra weight. You do not need to lift heavy weights all the time just to lose weight. Careful planning of your meal will also improve your goal to lose weight faster. This method of controlling your diet is also good for your health since it will give you more endurance in your daily exercises and work routine. If you do your exercise more than the usual plan that you have, you should also change your meal diet to fit the existing work to avoid stress and dehydration in your system.

A healthy meal plan for weight loss is your partner in your workouts; the more sweat you give out from your body also requires you to eat more healthy food to compensate for this kind of physical exertion. Less food in taking during a hard routine exercise is not a good idea. Make sure you balance your work and your diet to avoid body break down in the future. Just remember to take more fluids or liquid during a task to avoid dehydration.

During the planning of your healthy meal plans for weight loss, make sure that you check your doctors' consent and advice before any action to prevent any injuries in your workouts. There is a better meal plan for each person, so check the best meal or diet meal plan before you decided to hit the gym for some workouts. Remember that prevention is better than cure. Just be wise in your decision and plan about your healthy meal. You know what they say, better safe than sorry.

Maintaining a healthy body weight can be tough and losing weight a more difficult task. If you have tried to shed pounds before and were unsuccessful, you might think that meal plans do not work for you. There are plenty of simple but effective ways to avoid common meal planning blunders and achieve long-lasting weight loss success.

Here Are Some Helpful Tips For Meal Planning For Weight Loss

1. Plan Your Meal: Planning your meals helps you develop new health behaviors. Without preparation, you may always struggle with your diet and yo-yo-ing weight. Before rushing to the supermarket for your weekly shop, stop and take some time to plan out the upcoming week. Include healthy lunches and snacks that you can throw in a bag for your busiest days. Make sure you choose fresh and organic food as well as lean cuts of meat for the healthiest choices.

2. Healthy And Simple: Planning for your daily meals and snacks need not be complicated. Simple foods like fruits and nuts contain plenty of nutrients yet with less-calories which is best for your diet. Simple yet nutritious. There are plenty of websites that can help you plan nutritious, healthy and simple meals.

3. Plan Healthy Treats: Choose to be healthy by purchasing natural and healthy foods. Foods such as low-fat cheese, yogurt, veggies, and fresh fruit are great choices for a low-calorie diet. Keep this food readily available in your home and your workplace. As much as possible, avoid junk foods that have no nutritional value and only add calories to your diet.

4. Start With Breakfast: Starting your day with a healthy breakfast will boost your metabolism and save you from mindless nibbling and bingeing later on. Individuals who consume breakfast regularly tend to consume fewer calories throughout the day.

5. Prepare Your Meals Ahead: Preparing healthy meals ahead of time will help you stay motivated and you will have more control over your meals and snacks. This keeps you from buying unhealthy foods that often lead to overeating.

6. Drink More Water: Replacing soda, alcohol and other drinks with water will help you lose weight more because these drinks contain a high amount of calories which can disrupt you from achieving your goal. Water is essential for the body because it hydrates and aids in the fat-burning process.

7. Maintaining Weight Requires You To Practice A Healthy And Balanced Diet: To lose weight, you should consume fewer calories than you burn but do so with a healthy plan in mind. Meal planning for weight loss involves discipline and vital to be successful in your weight loss goal.

We have tried to elaborate below that what is a healthy diet meal plan through suggestions and tips so that you can manage this according to your needs and wishes.

1. The first step toward a healthy diet meal plan is to divide your meal in five to six smaller meals a day where each of the meals can be served one or two days at max.

2. Including healthy and delicious snacks in between the meals if you feel hunger.

3. Plan your meals for one week and there must be a variety of food and ingredients. You must plan your snacks as well before time.

4. Avoid junk food and chips, ice cream, sodas or colas, cookies, and chocolates.

5. Your healthy diet meal plan can include crackers, popcorn, fresh and dried fruit, yogurt, pretzels, baby carrots, low-fat cheese, peanut butter, air-popped popcorn cereals, and nuts and seeds.

6. Drink a lot of water in a day and especially before taking a meal. It will maintain the proper level of fluid in your body and will also make you less hungry.

7. Reduce the usage of fats and avoid using much milk, chicken, margarine or butter, mayonnaise, and use less oil in cooking your healthy diet meal planned.

8. Soft drinks and juices have a higher number of vitamins so avoid using these.

9. Add more grains in your food, as whole-grain loaves of bread can be used instead of white loaves of bread and brown rice instead of white rice.

10. Don't use the foods which have a high frequency of sugar and eat vegetables in each meal.

11. Never skip breakfast as it boosts your metabolisms and also decreases the hunger for the later day.

12. Eat very slowly and do not eat while doing something else. As eating while studying or watching television always noticed uncontrolled.

13. Collect several recipes and then categorize those in different types so that these could be used while making a diet meal plan.

14. When you will plan for simple meals it will help you have a wide range of foods and you will eat almost every healthy thing repeatedly in several ways.

15. You can also plan for a packed lunch which may be in the form of some good sandwiches. It will keep you away from any junk or fast food and you can also add a list of sandwich filling to change the taste regularly.

16. Try not to repeat the same meal on the same day and always use different foods in all meals.

17. Maintain good storage of healthy foods in your cabinets and refrigerator. Quick and simple meal ingredients and standbys will help you maintain your healthy diet meal plan.

18. A healthy diet meal plan in a week should have, two vegetarian meals, two meals using fish, one meal with poultry, and one meal with red meat.

19. Purchase a wide range of fruits and vegetables and serve plenty of vegetables in a meal.

20. Plan meals which also have healthy ways of cooking. No more fried foods.

21. You can also enjoy other favorite foods that have a larger number of calories in them but very less quantity and occasionally.

22. An exercise program should also be made along with your diet plan so that you can burn the extra calories.

23. Investigate what type of vitamins, minerals, and calories a food type provides and you can then use charting against the diet meat plan you made for yourself or your family.

CHAPTER 13 - EMOTIONAL EATING

What Does Emotional Eating Mean?

Emotional eating: Emotional eating is the practice of consuming large quantities of food -- usually "comfort" or junk foods -- in response to feelings instead of hunger. Experts estimate that 75% of overeating is caused by emotions

What Is Emotional Eating?

We don't always eat just to satisfy physical hunger. Many of us also turn to food for comfort, stress relief, or to reward ourselves. And when we do, we tend to reach for junk food, sweets, and other comforting but unhealthy foods. You might reach for a pint of ice cream when you're feeling down, order a pizza if you're bored or lonely, or swing by the drive-through after a stressful day at work. Emotional eating is using food to make yourself feel better—to fill emotional needs, rather than your stomach. Unfortunately, emotional eating doesn't fix emotional problems. It usually makes you feel worse. Afterward, not only does the original emotional issue remain, but you also feel guilty for overeating.

- ❖ Are you an emotional eater?
- ❖ Do you eat more when you're feeling stressed?
- ❖ Do you eat when you're not hungry or when you're full?
- ❖ Do you eat to feel better (to calm and soothe yourself when you're sad, mad, bored, anxious, etc.)?
- ❖ Do you reward yourself with food?
- ❖ Do you regularly eat until you've stuffed yourself?
- ❖ Does food make you feel safe? Do you feel like food is a friend?
- ❖ Do you feel powerless or out of control around food?

4 Types Of Eating

The 4 Types of Eating are fuel eating, joy eating, fog eating, and storm eating. Anytime you eat anything ever, you can categorize it into one of those four components, and by doing that, you can see where the extra overeating and the extra calories and the weight are coming from.

Why Food?

Negative emotions may lead to a feeling of emptiness or an emotional void. Food is believed to be a way to fill that void and create a false feeling of "fullness" or temporary wholeness.

Other Factors Include:

- ❖ Retreating from social support during times of emotional need
- ❖ Not engaging in activities that might otherwise relieve stress, sadness, and so on
- ❖ Not understanding the difference between physical and emotional hunger
- ❖ Using negative self-talking that's related to bingeing episodes. This can create a cycle of emotional eating
- ❖ Changing cortisol levels in response to stress, leading to cravings.

The Difference Between Emotional Hunger And Physical Hunger

Before you can break free from the cycle of emotional eating, you first need to learn how to distinguish between emotional and physical hunger. This can be trickier than it sounds, especially if you regularly use food to deal with your feelings.

Emotional hunger can be powerful, so it's easy to mistake it for physical hunger. But there are clues you can look for to help you tell physical and emotional hunger apart.

Emotional hunger comes on suddenly. It hits you in an instant and feels overwhelming and urgent. Physical hunger, on the other hand, comes on more gradually. The urge to eat doesn't feel as dire or demand instant satisfaction (unless you haven't eaten for a very long time).

Emotional hunger craves specific comfort foods. When you're physically hungry, almost anything sounds good—including healthy stuff like vegetables. But emotional hunger craves junk food or sugary snacks that provide an instant rush. You feel like you need cheesecake or pizza, and nothing else will do.

Emotional hunger often leads to mindless eating. Before you know it, you've eaten a whole bag of chips or an entire pint of ice cream without really paying attention or fully enjoying it. When you're eating in response to physical hunger, you're typically more aware of what you're doing.

Emotional hunger isn't satisfied once you're full. You keep wanting more and more, often eating until you're uncomfortably stuffed. Physical hunger, on the other hand, doesn't need to be stuffed. You feel satisfied when your stomach is full.

Emotional hunger isn't located in the stomach. Rather than a growling belly or a pang in your stomach, you feel your hunger as a craving you can't get out of your head. You're focused on specific textures, tastes, and smells.

Emotional hunger often leads to regret, guilt, or shame. When you eat to satisfy physical hunger, you're unlikely to feel guilty or ashamed because you're simply giving your body what it needs. If you feel guilty after you eat, it's likely because you know deep down that you're not eating for nutritional reasons.

Emotional hunger	Physical hunger
Emotional hunger comes on suddenly	Physical hunger comes on gradually
Emotional hunger feels like it needs to be satisfied instantly	Physical hunger can wait
Emotional hunger craves specific comfort foods	Physical hunger is open to options—lots of things sound good
Emotional hunger isn't satisfied with a full stomach	Physical hunger stops when you're full
Emotional eating triggers feelings of guilt, powerlessness, and shame	Eating to satisfy physical hunger doesn't make you feel bad about yourself

Identify Your Emotional Eating Triggers

The first step in putting a stop to emotional eating is identifying your triggers. What situations, places, or feelings make you reach for the comfort of food? Most emotional eating is linked to unpleasant feelings, but it can also be triggered by positive emotions, such as rewarding yourself for achieving a goal or celebrating a holiday or happy event.

Common Causes Of Emotional Eating

Stress: Ever notice how stress makes you hungry? It's not just in your mind. When stress is chronic, as it so often is in our chaotic, fast-paced world, your body produces high levels of the stress hormone, cortisol. Cortisol triggers cravings for salty, sweet, and fried foods—foods that give you a burst of energy and pleasure. The more uncontrolled stress in your life, the more likely you are to turn to food for emotional relief.

Stuffing Emotions: Eating can be a way to temporarily silence or "stuff down" uncomfortable emotions, including anger, fear, sadness, anxiety, loneliness, resentment, and shame. While you're numbing yourself with food, you can avoid the difficult emotions you'd rather not feel.

Boredom Or Feelings Of Emptiness: Do you ever eat simply to give yourself something to do, to relieve boredom, or as a way to fill a void in your life? You feel unfulfilled and empty, and food is a way to occupy your mouth and your time. At the moment, it fills you up and distracts you from underlying feelings of purposelessness and dissatisfaction with your life.

Childhood Habits: Think back to your childhood memories of food. Did your parents reward good behavior with ice cream, take you out for pizza when you got a good report card, or serve you, sweets, when you were feeling sad? These habits can often carry over into adulthood. Or your eating may be driven by nostalgia—for cherished memories of grilling burgers in the backyard with your dad or baking and eating cookies with your mom.

Social Influences: Getting together with other people for a meal is a great way to relieve stress, but it can also lead to overeating. It's easy to overindulge simply because the food is there or because everyone else is eating. You may also overeat in social situations out of nervousness. Or perhaps your family or circle of friends encourages you to overeat, and it's easier to go along with the group.

Emotional eating can sabotage your weight-loss efforts. It often leads to eating too much especially too much of high-calorie, sweet and fatty foods. The good news is that if you're prone to emotional eating, you can take steps to regain control of your eating habits and get back on track with your weight-loss goals.

How The Mood-Food-Weight Loss Cycle Works

Emotional eating is eating as a way to suppress or soothe negative emotions, such as stress, anger, fear, boredom, sadness, and loneliness. Major life events or, more commonly, the hassles of daily life can trigger negative emotions that lead to emotional eating and disrupt your weight-loss efforts. These triggers might include:

- ❖ Relationship conflicts
- ❖ Work or other stressors
- ❖ Fatigue
- ❖ Financial pressures
- ❖ Health problems

Although some people eat less in the face of strong emotions, if you're in emotional distress you might turn to impulsive or binge eating, quickly consuming whatever's convenient without enjoyment. Your emotions can become so tied to the eating habits that you automatically reach for a treat whenever you're angry or stressed without thinking about what you're doing.

Food also serves as a distraction. If you're worried about an upcoming event or stewing over a conflict, for instance, you may focus on eating comfort food instead of dealing with the painful situation.

Whatever emotions drive you to overeat, the result is often the same. The effect is temporary, the emotions return and you likely then bear the additional burden of guilt about setting back your weight-loss goal. This can also lead to an unhealthy cycle — your emotions trigger you to overeat, you beat yourself up for getting off your weight-loss track, you feel bad and you overeat again.

How Do You Get Back On Track?

When negative emotions threaten to trigger emotional eating, you can take steps to control cravings. To help stop emotional eating, try these tips:

1. Keep A Food Diary: Write down what you eat, how much you eat, when you eat, how you're feeling when you eat and how hungry you are. Over time, you might see patterns that reveal the connection between mood and food.

2. Tame Your Stress: If stress contributes to your emotional eating, try a stress management technique, such as yoga, meditation or deep breathing.

3. Have A Hunger Reality Check: Is your hunger physical or emotional? If you ate just a few hours ago and don't have a rumbling stomach, you're probably not hungry. Give the craving time to pass.

4. Get Support: You're more likely to give in to emotional eating if you lack a good support network. Lean on family and friends or consider joining a support group.

5. Fight Boredom: Instead of snacking when you're not hungry, distract yourself and substitute a healthier behavior. Take a walk, watch a movie, play with your cat, listen to music, read, surf the internet or call a friend.

6. Take Away Temptation: Don't keep hard-to-resist comfort foods in your home. And if you feel angry or blue, postpone your trip to the grocery store until you have your emotions in check.

7. Don't Deprive Yourself: When trying to lose weight, you might limit calories too much, eat the same foods repeatedly and banish treats. This may just serve to increase your food cravings, especially in response to emotions. Eat satisfying amounts of healthier foods, enjoy an occasional treat and get plenty of variety to help curb cravings.

8. Snack Healthy: If you feel the urge to eat between meals, choose a healthy snack, such as fresh fruit, vegetables with low-fat dip, nuts or unbuttered popcorn. Or try lower-calorie versions of your favorite foods to see if they satisfy your craving.

9. Learn From Setbacks: If you have an episode of emotional eating, forgive yourself and start fresh the next day. Try to learn from the experience and make a plan for how you can prevent it in the future. Focus on the positive changes you're making in your eating habits and give yourself credit for making changes that'll lead to better health.

10. Practice Willpower: Willpower is like a muscle you need to train, so the more you say no to cookies and yes to the gym, the easier those decisions become.

11. Focus On Health, Not Weight. It's Not About A Number On The Scale: Ten years ago I never would have believed I could feel this happy and healthy, but I do, and that makes it all worth it

12. Take It One Meal At A Time: If you mess up, don't beat yourself up over it. And instead of saying "I'll start fresh tomorrow" (which could get pretty out of hand if you "mess up" with a bagel and cream cheese in the morning), try "I'll start fresh with the next thing I eat."

Alternatives To Emotional Eating

If you're depressed or lonely, call someone who always makes you feel better, plays with your dog or cat, or look at a favorite photo or cherished memento.

If you're anxious, expend your nervous energy by dancing to your favorite song, squeezing a stress ball, or taking a brisk walk.

If you're exhausted, treat yourself with a hot cup of tea, take a bath, light some scented candles, or wrap yourself in a warm blanket.

If you're bored, read a good book, watch a comedy show, explore the outdoors, or turn to an activity you enjoy (woodworking, playing the guitar, shooting hoops, scrapbooking, etc.).

Pause when cravings hit and check-in with yourself

Most emotional eaters feel powerless over their food cravings. When the urge to eat hits, it's all you can think about. You feel an almost unbearable tension that demands to be fed, right now! Because you've tried to resist in the past and failed, you believe that your willpower just isn't up to snuff. But the truth is that you have more power over your cravings than you think.

Take 5 Before You Give In To A Craving

Emotional eating tends to be automatic and virtually mindless. Before you even realize what you're doing, you've reached for a tub of ice cream and polished off half of it. But if you can take a moment to pause and reflect when you're hit with a craving, you allow yourself to make a different decision.

- ❖ Can you put off eating for five minutes? Or just start with one minute. Don't tell yourself you can't give in to the craving; remember, the forbidden is extremely tempting. Just tell yourself to wait.

- ❖ While you're waiting, check-in with yourself. How are you feeling? What's going on emotionally? Even if you end up eating, you'll have a better understanding of why you did it. This can help you set yourself up for a different response next time.

- ❖ Learn to accept your feelings even the bad ones

- ❖ While it may seem that the core problem is that you're powerless over food, emotional eating stems from feeling powerless over your emotions. You don't feel capable of dealing with your feelings head-on, so you avoid them with food.

- ❖ Allowing yourself to feel uncomfortable emotions can be scary. You may fear that, like Pandora's box, once you open the door you won't be able to shut it. But the truth is that when we don't obsess over or suppress our emotions, even the most painful and difficult feelings subside relatively quickly and lose their power to control our attention.

To do this you need to become mindful and learn how to stay connected to your moment-to-moment emotional experience. This can enable you to rein in stress and repair emotional problems that often trigger emotional eating. HelpGuide's free Emotional Intelligence Toolkit can show you how.

Indulge Without Overeating By Savoring Your Food

When you eat to feed your feelings, you tend to do so quickly, mindlessly consuming food on autopilot. You eat so fast you miss out on the different tastes and textures of your food—as well as your body's cues that you're full and no longer hungry. But by slowing down and savoring every bite, you'll not only enjoy your food more but you'll also be less likely to overeat.

Slowing down and savoring your food is an important aspect of mindful eating, the opposite of mindless, emotional eating. Try taking a few deep breaths before starting your food, putting your utensils down between bites, and focusing on the experience of eating. Pay attention to the textures, shapes, colors, and smells of your food. How does each mouthful taste? How does it make your body feel? By slowing down in this way, you'll find you appreciate each bite of food much more. You can even indulge in your favorite foods and feel full on much less. It takes time for the body's fullness signal to reach your brain, so taking a few moments to consider how you feel after each bite hungry or satiated can help you avoid overeating.

Support Yourself With Healthy Lifestyle Habits

When you're physically strong, relaxed, and well-rested, you're better able to handle the curveballs that life inevitably throws your way. But when you're already exhausted and overwhelmed, any little hiccup has the potential to send you off the rails and straight toward the refrigerator. Exercise, sleep, and other healthy lifestyle habits will help you get through difficult times without emotional eating.

1. **Make Daily Exercise A Priority:** Physical activity does wonders for your mood and energy levels, and it's also a powerful stress reducer. And getting into the exercise habit is easier than you may think.

2. **Aim For 8 Hours Of Sleep Every Night:** When you don't get the sleep you need, your body craves sugary foods that will give you a quick energy boost. Getting plenty of rest will help with appetite control and reduce food cravings.

3. **Make Time For Relaxation:** Permit yourself to take at least 30 minutes every day to relax, decompress, and unwind. This is your time to take a break from your responsibilities and recharge your batteries.

4. **Connect With Others:** Don't underestimate the importance of close relationships and social activities. Spending time with positive people who enhance your life will help protect you from the negative effects of stress.

Keep An Emotional Eating Diary

You probably recognized yourself in at least a few of the previous descriptions. But even so, you'll want to get even more specific. One of the best ways to identify the patterns behind your emotional eating is to keep track of a food and mood diary.

Every time you overeat or feel compelled to reach for your version of comfort food Kryptonite, take a moment to figure out what triggered the urge. If you backtrack, you'll usually find an upsetting event that kicked off the emotional eating cycle. Write it all down in your food and mood diary: what you ate (or wanted to eat), what happened to upset you, how you felt before you ate, what you felt as you were eating, and how you felt afterward.

Over time, you'll see a pattern emerge. Maybe you always end up gorging yourself after spending time with a critical friend. Or perhaps you stress eat whenever you're on a deadline or when you attend family functions. Once you identify your emotional eating triggers, the next step is identifying healthier ways to feed your feelings.

When To Seek Professional Help

If you've tried self-help options but you still can't control emotional eating, consider therapy with a mental health professional. Therapy can help you understand why you eat emotionally and learn coping skills. Therapy can also help you discover whether you have an eating disorder, which can be connected to emotional eating.

CHAPTER 14 - FASTING WEIGHT LOSS

Fasting weight loss plans can be used for people who need to drop a few pounds in a short period. It is not unheard of for someone to drop 3-4 pounds a day on a fasting diet. Fasting should not be sustained for long periods. If the body does not receive the proper intake of nutrients, it will use what is available and begin to feed on itself.

Fasting for weight loss progressed over thousands of years as a religious ritual usually to honor one's God. Today, many adults and teenagers, are under a lot of pressure believing they must look like magazine models to be acceptable and they start fasting for weight loss. They can not be more wrong.

Losing weight is about determination. Improvement in self-confidence is an added benefit as your self-image improves. By fasting for weight loss you deprive your body of essential nutrients that need to be replenished daily. You're playing with fire. It's dangerous and not smart.

Fasting for weight loss prevents natural metabolic activities necessary for energy. Without this natural process, you will tire more easily. After fasting too long, you won't think properly and may become agitated. Many people have tried fasting to lose weight and have had major problems with it. Including body organ shutdown to even death. After long-term fasting, you may be surprised that the damage caused by fasting is irreversible. When you break your fasting you will probably be heavier than when you started. You will end up being disappointed, hungry and unwell. Remember, fasting is just losing water weight and not fat weight. It has been proven that fasting for weight loss is not the best solution to losing weight. Your best bet is to eat 4 to 6 small meals per day, do cardiovascular training and drink lots of water.

Fast Weight Loss Strategies

One effective strategy is a fast weight loss diet. Although there are lots of diet plans that are being advertised on the Internet that promise quick weight loss, it is still best to talk to your doctor regarding this. Your physician can provide you with the facts on weight loss and help you decide which weight loss supplement may be right for your situation. If possible, you should also eat foods in moderation and be more aware of your serving sizes.

Aside from diet, weight loss pills and supplements can also be effective. However, with the increasing supplement scams in the market these days, it can be very risky to try these products since a few of these are proven ineffective. This is why you must consult your physician before you take any weight loss pills or supplements.

The last strategy for weight loss is increased exercise. Exercise is considered the most important component of overall health and fitness. This is one weight-loss method that has never been banned, never been investigated, and never been included in a "weight loss scam" report. This is safe, effective, and brings many benefits to the body aside from weight loss. Though exercise may not give you fast results, it is a sure and proven method of weight loss.

These are the three effective strategies that can help you achieve quick weight loss results. When these three are combined, you are guaranteed to achieve your target healthy weight.

7 Fast Weight Loss Tips To Speed Up Metabolism

These fast weight loss tips will help you to drop a lot of extra pounds if you need to lose quite a bit of weight. These 7 fast weight loss tips will also help you, if you are already in decent physical condition, to sculpt your body to an even greater degree. Any weight loss tips to help speed up metabolism do just that. They help you. You still must have your overall fitness and nutrition plan in line with the goals you want to achieve. You need to be focused on each aspect of your plan. If you expect to use these fast weight loss tips but don't exercise and just watch television eating a bag of chips every night, they won't do a thing for you.

Are You Ready To Add These Fast Weight Loss Tips To Your Lifestyle?

To get rid of any amount of excess weight, you must speed up metabolism. Your metabolism is a biochemical process that occurs in your body. Your metabolism helps to break down nutrients in your bloodstream. This helps you to add more lean muscle, resulting in a greater expenditure of energy, meaning you'll get rid of more fat. You have billions of cells in your body that can use up an enormous amount of energy if you are active. The fast weight loss tips listed below will help you do this. However, if you aren't active they won't burn up much at all, meaning you'll tend to easily add fat to your body.

Thankfully, using the fast weight loss tips in conjunction with your healthy and active lifestyle you can speed up your metabolism quite noticeably.

Fast Weight Loss Tips: 1. Eat Specific Foods: Several food additives, like spices, can help to speed up your metabolism by creating a thermodynamic burn that has been shown to last a few hours after you eat.

Fast Weight Loss Tips: 2. Time Your Meals: The majority of your calories should be earlier in the day. Your meals should contain less total calories as the day goes on. Try to eat little or preferably nothing at all after your evening meal. Don't skip any meals. You should be eating 4 - 6 meals each day.

Fast Weight Loss Tips: 3. Make Sure You Eat Enough: One of the biggest mistakes people make when trying to lose weight is they don't eat enough. If you don't consume the proper amount of calories you will send your body into what is known as a survival mode. This happens when your body does not have enough calories, so it conserves energy to prepare for possible starvation. On the opposite side of this, is if you eat too many calories the excess will be stored as fat. You need to exercise to burn more calories than you eat. Therefore, moderation is key when it comes to calorie intake.

Fast Weight Loss Tips: 4. Increase Your Daily Activities: To prevent fat storage and to drop any excess that you might be carrying you must increase your daily activities. This needs to include weight training and cardiovascular training. The more calories you burn, the faster you will lose weight. It's that simple. An increase in lean muscle mass results in a dramatic increase in fat burning. One more thing; try to exercise first thing in the morning. Research has shown that you can dramatically increase your fat-burning ability if you exercise after a fasted state. Meaning just after you wake up.

Fast Weight Loss Tips: 5. Do Weight Lifting Before Doing Any Cardiovascular Work: The only exception, of course, is to perform 5 - 10 minutes of cardio before your weight training to warm up your muscles. This is important because you need the energy in your muscles for weight training. By the time your weight training session is complete, you will have used up all of your preferred energy sources. This means that you will be burning fat cells during your cardio session.

Here's What Happens If You Do This In Reverse

First, you will only be burning carbohydrate sources of energy during your cardiovascular workout. No fat cells will be used up for energy. Next, you will not have the energy in your muscles to get the most out of your weight training. You will not be able to increase your lean muscle, which is very important if you want to lose your excess weight.

Fast Weight Loss Tips: 6. Change Up Your Exercise Routine Regularly: For the most part, you should change some aspect of your workout every 2 - 3 weeks. This can be anything from the number of reps or sets per exercise. The exercise order you perform and the exercises themselves. If you do the same thing week after week, month after month your body will start to get used to what you're doing to it and will eventually stop making changes. You will also stop adding any more lean muscle. The more muscle you have the more calories you will burn even when at rest.

Fast Weight Loss Tips: 7. Meal Combinations. Always Eat Protein/Carbohydrate Meals Earlier In The Day: Eat protein/fat combination meals (meaning little to no carbohydrates) in the late afternoon and evening. The only exception is if you normally exercise in the evening. Then your first meal after your workout should consist of protein and carbohydrates. Never eat carbohydrates and fat together in the same meal. With these seven fast weight loss tips, you will speed up metabolism and burn excess body fat at a much faster rate.

Try these fast weight loss tips out for a while and you'll notice a difference after a couple of weeks.

Fast Weight Loss - Importance Of Boosting Metabolism

There are many weight loss programs and weight loss products to help you attain fast weight loss if you are somebody that has struggled with weight issues all your life. If they do not provide ways and discuss the importance of boosting metabolism, prepare to fail. This article discusses metabolism and a few facts about metabolism to get you on the right track to achieving fast weight loss. Fast weight loss is achieved when more calories are burned per day than the number of calories that are consumed per day. Your metabolic rate is the number of calories that you burn per day. Some people have a fast metabolism and may not struggle with weight as much as someone with a slow metabolism. Metabolism implies all the activity in the body including converting food into energy, creation of hormones and enzymes, muscle creation and/or repair, etc. It is affected by various factors including genes, age, lifestyle, etc.

1. Skipping Meals Or Eating Little

Most people think that if they simply stop eating, they will lose weight. What usually happens is that the body goes into starvation mode and starts storing food including fat. Also, starvation cannot realistically be sustained in the long run to lose weight fast. What also happens when this food is being stored as the body goes into starvation mode, is that metabolism is slowed down to allow more fat to be stored. Starving yourself or consuming low-calorie products will not work in the long run to help you achieve and maintain fast weight loss. Eating frequent meals and not skipping breakfast especially, will keep your metabolism working to enable you to lose weight fast.

2. Managing Insulin Levels

When sugars and carbohydrates are consumed, the body converts them to glucose which is then released into the bloodstream. The pancreas then produces insulin to remove this glucose from the blood and distribute it to the different cells in the body that need it for energy. When there are an excessive amount and consumption of foods that mainly produce energy such as carbohydrates, insulin will be secreted in greater amounts and the insulin will store the excess carbs as glycogen in the muscles, liver and circulatory system to be used as needed when blood glucose levels decrease. Any excess carbs that can not be stored as glycogen are converted into fat and then stored in the body's fatty tissues. When the body produces excess insulin due to the heightened levels of glucose in the blood, weight problems as well as being at risk of developing chronic diseases arise. This mainly occurs because of the kind of food being eaten. Eating refined foods such as white rice and white bread does not put the metabolism to work which increases blood sugar levels.

Consuming complex carbohydrates which include none of the "white" foods and more whole grains puts the metabolism to work and reduces blood sugar levels and the need for excessive amounts of insulin. When you consume the "white" foods which lead to increased blood glucose levels, the insulin will overreact in an attempt to remove the excess glucose from the blood which leads to a drop in the blood sugar which usually causes people to feel hungry a lot quicker for more of the bad carbs leading to a repeat of this unhealthy process. This cycle can continue until finally, the body becomes insulin resistant which leads to the accumulation of insulin in the blood which is then expelled from the body through urine. This leaves the body without the energy that it desperately needs to properly function leading to various chronic diseases and complications.

3. Physical Activity

Physical activity is required for fast weight loss that can be maintained on a long term basis. Physical activity can boost metabolism leading to more calories being burned per day and allow you to lose weight fast. If you lead a sedentary lifestyle, you will gain weight. Simple as that unless you happen to be one of the lucky few with a hyperactive metabolic rate. If you do not incorporate physical activity into your weight loss program, you will not enjoy any of the benefits of fast weight loss that can be gotten by incorporating physical activity into your weight loss program. To boost your metabolism, you should exercise for at least thirty minutes, at least three times a week and be consistent for optimal benefits that include fast weight loss.

CONCLUSION

Hypnosis for weight loss, what can it do for you? There are many things hypnosis can do beyond weight reduction. Some of these include improved motivation to lose weight, increased self-discipline, along with the willpower that is required to lose weight. Hypnosis for weight loss will remove the mental blocks a person has to lose weight. Some of the additional benefits of using hypnosis for weight reduction and intuitive eating include.

- ❖ The truth behind loss weight
- ❖ How to start loss weight safely and effectively
- ❖ Benefits to expect
- ❖ Different types of foods to be eating for weight loss
- ❖ Foods and meal plans to help make your fast easier
- ❖ Exercises to encourage weight-loss while fasting and eating

Hypnosis for weight loss is one tool that people are using more and more to try and get back into a healthy lifestyle. For many people, this sounds like a great idea, but they are not even sure how something like this would work. Here is a brief overview of how hypnosis for weight loss works.

Like all hypnosis plans, the goal is to change how the subconscious works. Training your subconscious will make changes to the way you think and the way you act, catapulting you to making positive changes in your life. I think most people are familiar with using hypnosis for quitting bad habits like drinking and smoking. By changing the subconscious, the desire and the need for those things lessen, making you able to control your urges. The same basic principals from those procedures are being used for weight loss hypnosis

However, if hypnosis for weight loss is coupled with some other normal workouts and diet plans for slimming down, it can provide better results. Hypnosis provides you with an advanced state of consciousness in which concentration levels are higher. In such a state mind, you will be keener and more receptive to suggestions. Therefore, hypnosis helps make the person-focused and oriented to the concept of shedding pounds. Whether you are looking into hypnosis for weight loss or fear of flying, you can succeed. Hypnosis allows you to try new things in a controlled environment. You can practice new behaviors before actually engaging in them. If you are looking to get control over your behavior and your life in general, give hypnosis a try.

The goal of this beginner's guide is to provide everything you need to know about hypnosis in loss weight .

Part Two

Introduction

Weight loss can be a challenging and overwhelming journey. Many weight loss resources focus largely on your diet, which is certainly important but can also be overwhelming. When you embark on the journey of weight loss, you might find yourself struggling to step away from old habits that lead to your weight gain in the first place. You may find yourself constantly bouncing back and forth between being "on the wagon" and "off the wagon," which may lead to you feeling guilty and struggling even more to fulfill your desires of weight loss.

Many times, what people do not realize is that your diet is only *partially* responsible for your ability to lose weight. Your mindset accounts for a big portion of your weight loss success. In fact, some might even argue that it is *more* important for you to master your mindset than anything else because, with the right mindset, you can set yourself up to accomplish anything. With that being said, when it comes to something such as weight loss, a simple shift in your mindset is unlikely to be enough. You will likely need a full mindset makeover to help you commit to your new weight loss journey and stay on track. That is where hypnosis comes in.

As you will learn, hypnosis is a powerful practice that allows you to essentially tap into your subconscious mind and begin to rewire your mindset. This means that you are not just changing your thoughts on a conscious level, but you are changing them right down to the very root of what encourages your thoughts in the first place. For many people, this is the difference between successful weight loss and unsuccessful weight loss. If you have been struggling with yo-yo dieting, feelings of defeat and general overwhelm when it comes to weight loss, hypnosis is likely exactly what you need to help you get your whole mind on board with your transformation.

When you change your mind, right down to the very way that it is wired, you change the entire way that you interact with food. You completely shift your habits around what inspires you to eat, what you choose to eat, and even how your body digests that food. Through these transformations, you find yourself experiencing healthy and natural weight loss in a way that does *not* feel like you are starving yourself or depriving yourself in order to reach your goals. Furthermore, these transformations are long-lasting as they truly do change the way your mind works. Plus, if you ever find yourself backsliding into old habits, you can indulge in your hypnosis as many times as you need to reinforce your changes and inspire your new habits once more.

If you are ready to change your approach to weight loss for good, it is time to lay a foundation that will actually work. I encourage you to start by reading this book in order so that you get exactly what you need—when you need it. However, I encourage you to also take a look at the 300 affirmations you have been provided with right away and keep some of them handy so that you can use these affirmations to inspire you to stay on track. You may wish to use the same affirmations over and over again, or change which ones you are using based on what you need in each situation.

Lastly, I want to let you know that all of the hypnosis practices described in this book are designed to be self-hypnosis. This means that you are the one in control over your hypnosis practices and that you, and you alone, are in control of how this works for your mind. This book is merely your guide to help walk you through the process, and nothing more. If you begin engaging in a hypnosis session and decide that you need to awaken yourself for any reason, simply open your eyes and go about your day as normal. With that being said, please make sure that you do not practice hypnosis when you are driving, operating heavy machinery, or otherwise engaging in activities that require your conscious awareness. Instead, practice it only when you can sit or lie down comfortably and without distraction for as long as you need to help you get the benefits of your meditation. This way, you are not at risk of becoming too relaxed to perform tasks you might need to perform, and you truly get the most out of each and every meditation session you engage in.

If you are ready to embark on your journey of natural weight loss using the power of hypnosis, it is time to begin! Please, take your time and keep an open mind when it comes to working through the pages of this book. I feel you will be thoroughly impressed and delightfully surprised by just how powerful hypnosis can be, and by how much it will transform your weight loss journey. Enjoy!

Chapter 1: Hypnosis for Rapid Weight Loss

Hypnosis is a powerful state of consciousness in which a person is able to essentially bypass their conscious thinking mind and tap into their subconscious thinking mind. Most of your habits and behaviours are formed in your subconscious thinking mind, so being able to tap into this part of your brain means that you can resolve the root cause of any unwanted habits or behaviours that are no longer serving you. Often, the roots of your habits and behaviours are formed without your conscious awareness or intention, which can lead to issues in your ability to actually overcome these habits or behaviours. Because you may not be clear on why they started, when, or how, you may struggle to understand them and find an effective resolve that helps you get past these behaviours. Hypnosis is a powerful method that can help you accomplish just that.

Hypnosis itself has been used for many different things, ranging from overcoming addictions or habits to helping people increase their sense of self-esteem and self-confidence. In some cases, people will even use hypnosis and guided visualization as a way to relax their mind or take a small break from the stresses of their day to day lives. In many ways, these "mini-vacations" are similar to daydreaming, except that they tend to be more structured and intentional.

When it comes to weight loss, hypnosis can be beneficial in many ways. From helping you change the way you think about food, to helping you change your actual behaviours around food, there are many things that can be accomplished with hypnosis. In this chapter, we are going to discover why hypnosis is so powerful, how it works for weight loss, and what you can do to help yourself lose weight using hypnosis.

How Hypnosis Works

Hypnosis is not what many people think it is. Because of old movies and performers, many people tend to think that hypnosis is some form of party trick that results in people struggling to have any control over themselves and their behaviours. This is actually not at all true. When you are engaging in hypnosis, you always remain in control of yourself, your body, and your behaviours. The suggestions being offered to you in guided meditations, such as the ones you will follow in this book, are just that: suggestions. Because hypnosis is not the absolute power that many movies depict it as it can take a few tries with hypnosis before you get the results you are looking for out of it. Many people will use about 3-4 sessions per area of focus in order to start seeing significant results. Some people may use up to 8-10 sessions before they experience absolute resolve of the issue that leads them to seek out the power of hypnosis in the first place.

When you are engaged in a hypnosis session, you are essentially relaxing to the point where you can sink deeper into your awareness. Think of this as being similar to dreaming without actually being asleep. Through this deep state of relaxation and the ability to sink into your deeper awareness, you are able to take suggestions from guided meditations and essentially rewire your subconscious mind. A great example of this is when people use self-hypnosis as a way to encourage themselves to increase their self-esteem. In this case, they are introducing positive thoughts about self-esteem and self-confidence into their subconscious minds so that they can begin to have a new mental experience around the topic of themselves.

As you "awaken" into your subconscious mind and introduce these new thoughts, you give your brain the opportunity to completely change how it works. Now, rather than your subconscious mind feeding your conscious mind unhelpful thoughts and perspectives, your subconscious mind will feed your conscious mind, helpful thoughts, and different perspectives that support your preferred reality. For example, with your self-esteem, this could result in you having thoughts that reinforce your self-esteem and a reality that fosters a deeper sense of self-esteem.

When it comes to your weight loss goals, your primary focus is on changing your subconscious mind around food. This way, you can eliminate any habits or behaviours that lead to compulsive eating, cravings, or overeating, and you can begin to instil new habits and behaviours on a subconscious level. What ends up happening is that when you awaken into your reality, you notice that you no longer have such strong cravings or urges around food, and you are able to have more pleasant and positive experiences with your diet.

Creating these changes on a subconscious level means that you are able to have an entirely renewed perspective around food and weight loss. Now, rather than depriving yourself, growing frustrated with cravings, or feeling defeated by your diets, you can feel confident and in alignment with your changes. Instead of having to fight off urges within yourself, you simply will not have them to begin with. This may seem too good to be true, but once you begin to engage in hypnosis and experience the changes in your subconscious mind, you will see just how powerful hypnosis actually is.

The Benefits of Hypnotherapy for Weight Loss

It is hard to pinpoint the single best benefit that comes from using hypnosis as a way to engage in weight loss. Hypnosis is a natural, lasting, and deeply impactful weight loss habit that you can use to completely change the way you approach weight loss, and food in general, for the rest of your life.

With hypnosis, you are not ingesting anything that results in hypnosis working. Instead, you are simply listening to guided hypnosis meditations that help you transform the way your subconscious mind works. As you change the way your subconscious mind works, you will find yourself not even having cravings or unhealthy food urges in the first place. This means no more fighting against your desires, yo-yo dieting, "falling off the wagon," or experiencing any inner conflict around your eating patterns, or your weight loss exercises that are helping you lose the weight. Instead, you will begin to have an entirely new mindset and perspective around weight loss that leads to you having more success in losing weight and keeping it off for good.

In addition to hypnosis itself being effective, you can also combine hypnosis with any other weight loss strategy you are using. Changed dietary behaviours, exercise routines, any medications you may be taking with the advisement of your medical practitioner, and any other weight loss practices you may be engaging in can all safely be done with hypnosis. By including hypnosis in your existing weight loss routines, you can improve your effectiveness and rapidly increase the success you experience in your weight loss patterns.

Finally, hypnosis can be beneficial for many things beyond weight loss. One of the side effects that you will likely notice once you start using hypnosis to help change your weight loss experience is that you also experience a boost in your confidence, self-esteem, and general feelings of positivity. Many people who use hypnosis on a regular basis find themselves feeling more positive and in better spirits in general. This means that not only will you lose weight, but you will also feel incredible and will have a happy and positive mood as well.

Examples of Effective Hypnosis Sessions

There are countless examples of when and where hypnosis has been effective in helping people with changing their lives, such as through changing their ability to lose weight. In one incredible example on PubMed, the US National Library of Medicine National Institutes of Health, *Kirsch L* discovered that using hypnosis to enhance cognitive-behavioral weight loss practices nearly doubled the effectiveness of other weight loss routines. This study was titled *Hypnotic Enhancement of Cognitive-Behavioral Weight Loss Treatments – Another Meta-Reanalysis.* This means that by using hypnosis in conjunction with a healthy diet and consistent exercise routine, you can possibly double your weight loss results, leading to faster and more effective weight loss.

Another study done by the same organization with *Bolocofsky DN, Spinler D,* and *Coulthard-Morris L* showed that hypnosis not only helped people lose weight but also helped them keep it off. This study, titled *Effectiveness of Hypnosis as an Adjunct to Behavioral Weight Management,* showed that over a two-year period, those who used hypnosis lost their desired amount of weight and kept it off. Alternatively, those who did not use hypnosis found little to no changes with their weight, and those who did struggled to keep the weight off.

Each of these studies proves that hypnosis is highly effective for both weight loss and weight management. So, how can you tell if a session was effective or not? Easy: you wait and see what happens after the session. Usually, people who undergo a hypnosis session report that they feel incredibly different immediately following the session. It is not uncommon for them to experience near-perfect changes for the hours following their session, or sometimes even the days following their session. After these initial changes, the individual will begin to experience a "regression." This is essentially where some of the change reverses, and they fall back into old patterns. This is because your subconscious is wired over several bouts of repetition, and so far, you have had plenty of repetition of your *old* patterns, not your *new* patterns.

Many people will mistakenly judge this regression as being evidence that the hypnosis did not work, but actually, it is just a natural symptom of being in the early stages of subconscious change. When this regression begins, you should start your next hypnosis session. The more that you engage in these hypnosis sessions each time you notice regression, the more effectively your subconscious mind will begin to change and maintain those changes for the long haul. At first, it may feel like you need to do your hypnosis sessions on a constant basis to really adapt to these changes. However, as you continually use them, you will find that it takes longer and longer for your regressions to happen and that they do not last nearly as long as they did previously. This is because your habits and behaviors are truly beginning to change on a subconscious level.

So, in order to gauge how effective a session has been, you ultimately need to gauge how you feel immediately following the session. If you feel inspired to change your behaviors, and it does not feel like an intense inner battle or struggle to do so, your hypnosis session has worked. If not, you may need to repeat the session once or twice to create that initial change. Then, over time, you will realize that you rely on the hypnosis less and less as these changes begin to become more lasting and permanent in your subconscious mind.

Step by Step: How You Will Lose Weight with Hypnosis

Losing weight with hypnosis works just like any other change with hypnosis will. However, it is important to understand the step by step process so that you know exactly what to expect during your weight loss journey with the support of hypnosis. In general, there are about seven steps that are involved with weight loss using hypnosis. The first step is when you decide to change; the second step involves your sessions; the third and fourth are your changed mindset and behaviors, the fifth step involves your regressions, the sixth is your management routines, and the seventh is your lasting change. To give you a better idea of what each of these parts of your journey looks like, let's explore them in greater detail below.

In your first step toward achieving weight loss with hypnosis, you have decided that you desire change and that you are willing to try hypnosis as a way to change your approach to weight loss. At this point, you are aware of the fact that you want to lose weight, and you have been shown the possibility of losing weight through hypnosis. This is likely the stage you are in right now as you begin reading this very book. You may find yourself feeling curious, open to trying something new, and a little bit skeptical as to whether or not this is actually going to work for you. You may also be feeling frustrated, overwhelmed, or even defeated by the lack of success you have seen using other weight loss methods, which may be what lead you to seek out hypnosis in the first place. At this stage, the best thing you can do is practice keeping an open and curious mind, as this is how you can set yourself up for success when it comes to your actual hypnosis sessions.

Your sessions account for stage two of the process. Technically, you are going to move from stage two through to stage five several times over before you officially move into stage six. Your sessions are the stage where you actually engage in hypnosis, nothing more and nothing less. During your sessions, you need to maintain your open mind and stay focused on how hypnosis can help you. If you are struggling to stay open-minded or are still skeptical about how this might work, you can consider switching from absolute confidence that it will help to have curiosity about how it might help instead.

Following your sessions, you are first going to experience a changed mindset. This is where you start to feel far more confident in your ability to lose weight and in your ability to keep the weight off. At first, your mindset may still be shadowed by doubt, but as you continue to use hypnosis and see your results, you will realize that it is entirely possible for you to create success with hypnosis. As these pieces of evidence start to show up in your own life, you will find your hypnosis sessions becoming even more powerful and even more successful.

In addition to a changed mindset, you are going to start to see changed behaviors. They may be smaller at first, but you will find that they increase over time until they reach the point where your behaviors reflect exactly the lifestyle you have been aiming to have. The best part about these changed behaviors is that they will not feel forced, nor will they feel like you have had to encourage yourself to get here: your changed mindset will make these changed behaviors incredibly easy for you to choose. As you continue working on your hypnosis and experiencing your changed mind, you will find that your behavioral changes grow more significant and more effortless every single time.

Following your hypnosis and your experiences with changed mindset and behaviors, you are likely going to experience regression periods. Regression periods are characterized by periods of time where you begin to engage in your old mindset and behavior once again. This happens because you have experienced this old mindset and behavioral patterns so many times over that they continue to have deep roots in your subconscious mind. The more you uproot them and reinforce your new behaviors with consistent hypnosis sessions, the more success you will have in eliminating these old behaviors and replacing them entirely with new ones. Anytime you experience the beginning of a regression period; you should set aside some time to engage in a hypnosis session to help you shift your mindset back into the state that you want and need it to be in.

Your management routines account for the sixth step, and they come into place after you have effectively experienced significant and lasting change from your hypnosis practices. At this point, you are not going to need to schedule as frequent of hypnosis sessions because you are experiencing such significant changes in your mindset. However, you may still want to do hypnosis sessions on a fairly consistent basis to ensure that your mindset remains changed and that you do not revert into old patterns. Sometimes, it can take up to 3-6 months or longer with these consistent management routine hypnosis sessions to maintain your changes and prevent you from experiencing a significant regression in your mindset and behavior.

The final step in your hypnosis journey is going to be the step where you come upon lasting changes. At this point, you are unlikely to need to schedule hypnosis sessions any longer. You should not need to rely on hypnosis at all to change your mindset because you have experienced such significant changes already, and you no longer find yourself regressing into old behaviors. With that being said, you may find that from time to time, you need to have a hypnosis session just to maintain your changes, particularly when an unexpected trigger may arise that may cause you to want to regress your behaviors. These unexpected changes can happen for years following your successful changes, so staying on top of them and relying on your healthy coping method of hypnosis is important as it will prevent you from experiencing a significant regression later in life.

Using Hypnosis to Encourage Healthy Eating and Discourage Unhealthy Eating

As you go through using hypnosis to support you with weight loss, there are a few ways that you are going to do so. One of the ways is, obviously, to focus on weight loss itself. Another way, however, is to focus on topics surrounding weight loss. For example, you can use hypnosis to help you encourage yourself to eat healthy while also helping discourage yourself from unhealthy eating. Effective hypnosis sessions can help you bust cravings for foods that are going to sabotage your success while also helping you feel more drawn to making choices that are going to help you effectively lose weight.

Many people will use hypnosis as a way to change their cravings, improve their metabolism, and even help themselves acquire a taste for eating healthier foods. You may also use this to help encourage you to develop the motivation and energy to actually prepare healthier foods and eat them so that you are more likely to have these healthier options available for you. If cultivating the motivation for preparing and eating healthy foods has been problematic for you, this type of hypnosis focus can be incredibly helpful.

Using Hypnosis to Encourage Healthy Lifestyle Changes

In addition to helping you encourage yourself to eat healthier while discouraging yourself from eating unhealthy foods, you can also use hypnosis to help encourage you to make healthy lifestyle changes. This can support you with everything from exercising more frequently to picking up more active hobbies that support your wellbeing in general.

You may also use this to help you eliminate hobbies or experiences from your life that may encourage unhealthy dietary habits in the first place. For example, if you tend to binge eat when you are stressed out, you might use hypnosis to help you navigate stress more effectively so that you are less likely to binge eat when you are feeling stressed out. If you tend to eat when you are feeling emotional or bored, you can use hypnosis to help you change those behaviors, too.

Hypnosis can be used to change virtually any area of your life that motivates you to eat unhealthily or otherwise neglect self-care to the point where you are sabotaging yourself from healthy weight loss. It truly is an incredibly versatile practice that you can rely on that will help you with weight loss, as well as help you with creating a healthier lifestyle in general. With hypnosis, there are countless ways that you can improve the quality of your life, making it an incredibly helpful practice for you to rely on. In the following chapters, we are going to explore how you can use hypnosis as a way to support you with weight loss, as well as improving your wellbeing overall.

Chapter 2: Meditation to Burn Fat

Before you can begin using meditations to do things such as help you burn fat, you need to make sure that you set yourself up properly for your meditation sessions. Each meditation is going to consist of you entering a deep state of relaxation, following a guided hypnosis, and then awakening yourself out of this state of relaxation. If done properly, you will find yourself experiencing the stages of changed mindset and changed behavior that follows the session.

In order to properly set yourself up for a meditation experience, you need to make sure that you have a quiet space where you can engage in your meditation. You want to be as uninterrupted as possible so that you do not stir awake from your meditation session. Aside from having a quiet space, you should also make sure that you are comfortable in the space that you will be in. For some of the meditations, I will share, you can be lying down or doing this meditation before bed so that the information sinks in as you sleep. For others, you are going to want to be sitting upright, ideally with your legs crossed on the floor, or with your feet planted on the floor as you sit in a chair. Staying in a sitting position, especially during morning meditations, will help you stay awake and increase your motivation. Laying down during these meditations earlier in the day may result in you draining your energy and feeling completely exhausted, rather than motivated. As a result, you may actually work *against* what you are trying to achieve.

Each of these meditations is going to involve a visualization practice; however, if you find that visualization is generally difficult for you, you can simply listen. The key here is to make sure that you keep as open of a mind as possible so that you can stay receptive to the information coming through these guided meditations.

Aside from all of the above, listening to low music, using a pillow or a small blanket, and dressing in comfortable loose clothing will all help you have better meditations. You want to make sure that you make these experiences the best possible so that you look forward to them and regularly engage in them. As well, the more relaxed and comfortable you are, the more receptive you will be to the information being provided to you within each meditation.

A Simple Daily Weight Loss Meditation

This meditation is an excellent simple meditation for you to use on a daily basis. It is a short meditation that will not take more than about 15 minutes to complete, and it will provide you with excellent motivation to stick to your weight loss regimen every single day. You should schedule time in your morning routine to engage in this simple daily weight loss meditation every single day. You can also complete it periodically throughout the day if you find your motivation dwindling or your mindset regressing. Over time, you should find that using it just once per day is plenty.

Because you are using this meditation in the morning, make sure that you are sitting upright with a straight spine so that you are able to stay engaged and awake throughout the entire meditation. Laying down or getting too comfortable may result in you feeling more tired, rather than more awake, from your meditation. Ideally, this meditation should lead to boosted energy as well as improved fat burning abilities within your body.

The Meditation

Start by gently closing your eyes and drawing your attention to your breath. As you do, I want you to track the next five breaths, gently and intentionally lengthening them to help you relax as deeply as you can. With each breath, breathe in to the count of five and out to the count of seven. Starting with your next breath in, one, two, three, four, five, and out, one, two, three, four, five, six, seven. Again, one, two, three, four, five, and out, one, two, three, four, five, six, seven. Breathe in, one, two, three, four, five, and breathe out, one, two, three, four, five, six, seven. Again, breathe in, one, two, three, four, five, and breathe out, one, two, three, four, five, six, seven. One more time, breathe in, one, two, three, four, five, and breathe out, one, two, three, four, five, six, seven.

Now that you are starting to feel more relaxed, I want you to draw your awareness into your body. First, become aware of your feet. Feel your feet relaxing deeply, as you visualize any stress or worry melting away from your feet. Now, become aware of your legs. Feel any stress or worry melting away from your legs as they begin to relax completely. Next, become aware of your glutes and pelvis, allowing any stress or worry to simply fade away as they completely relax. Now, become aware of your entire torso, allowing any stress or worry to melt away from your torso as it relaxes completely. Next, become aware of your shoulders, arms, hands, and fingers. Allow the stress and worry to melt away from your shoulders, arms, hands, and fingers as they relax completely. Now, let the stress and worry melt away from your neck, head, and face. Feel your neck, head, and face relaxing as any stress or worry melts away completely.

As you deepen into this state of relaxation, I want you to take a moment to visualize the space in front of you. Imagine that in front of you, you are standing there looking back at yourself. See every inch of your body as it is right now standing before you, casually, as you simply observe yourself. While you do, see what parts of your body you want to reduce fat in so that you can create a healthier, stronger body for yourself. Visualize the fat in these areas of your body, slowly fading away as you begin to carve out a healthier, leaner, and stronger body underneath. Notice how effortlessly this extra fat melts away as you continue to visualize yourself becoming a healthier and more vivacious version of yourself.

Now, I want you to visualize what this healthier, leaner version of yourself would be doing. Visualize yourself going through your typical daily routine, except from the perspective of your healthier self. What would you be eating? When and how would you be exercising? What would you spend your time doing? How do you feel about yourself? How different do you feel when you interact with the people around you, such as your family and your co-workers? What does life feel like when you are a healthier, leaner version of you?

Spend several minutes visualizing how different your life is now that your fat has melted away. Feel how natural it is for you to enjoy these healthier foods, and how easy it is for you to moderate your cravings and indulgences when you choose to treat yourself. Notice how easy it is for you to engage in exercise and how exercise feels enjoyable and like a wonderful hobby, rather than a chore that you have to force yourself to commit to every single day. Feel yourself genuinely enjoying life far more, all because the unhealthy fats that were weighing you down and disrupting your health have faded away. Notice how easy it was for you to get here, and how easy it is for you to continue to maintain your health and wellness as you continue to choose better and better choices for you and your body.

Feel how much you respect your body when you make these healthier choices, and how much you genuinely care about yourself. Notice how each meal and each exercise feels like an act of self-care, rather than a chore you are forcing yourself to engage in. Feel how good it feels to do something *for you.* For your wellbeing.

When you are ready, take that visualization of yourself and send the image out really far, watching it become nothing more than a spec in your field of awareness. Then, send it out into the ether, trusting that your subconscious mind will hold onto this vision of yourself and work daily on bringing this version of you into your current reality.

Now, awaken back into your body where you sit right now. Feel yourself feeling more motivated, more energized, and more excited about engaging in the activities that are going to improve your health and help you burn your fat. As you prepare to go about your day, hold onto that visualization and those feelings that you had of yourself, and trust that you can have this wonderful experience in your life. You can do it!

Fat Burning Meditation

This fat-burning meditation is a simple 30-minute meditation that is going to allow you to spend time visualizing your fat cells, reducing into smaller and smaller cells until they essentially vanish. Focusing on these types of hypnosis, meditations are said to help direct your subconscious mind on how to interact with your body so that you can begin to have a healthier and healthier body. When you focus on intentionally drawing your subconscious awareness into these activities, it encourages it to continue engaging in these activities on its own, even when you are not engaged in your hypnosis session.

This is a great meditation to engage in during the day anywhere from one to three times per week, or at bedtime. They say that meditating right before you fall asleep can be particularly potent, as you are meditating during a time where your subconscious mind is particularly active, and your conscious mind is already beginning to fall asleep. During this time, you are most likely to experience the level of relaxation and receptivity that is needed for your subconscious mind to really digest the changes that you are seeking to make within it.

The Meditation

To begin this meditation, allow yourself to close your eyes and begin to fade into a deep state of relaxation. Feel yourself relaxing deeper and deeper with each breath, and notice yourself falling into a lovely state of calmness. In order to help you deepen your relaxation, I am going to guide you through a practice that will take you to the deepest level of relaxation possible. To do this, I want you to visualize yourself standing at the top of a set of stairs. As I count down from ten to one, I want you to visualize yourself walking down that flight of stairs, taking just one step at a time. With each step you take, visualize yourself relaxing deeper and deeper until you find yourself in a deep state of relaxation and ready to engage in a hypnotic visualization session.

Beginning with ten, visualize yourself taking a step down the stairs. Notice your surroundings, including the color of the walls, what the bottom step looks like, and any decorations that may be surrounding you. With nine, step down again, and see yourself getting closer to the bottom of the flight of stairs. Notice your relaxation doubling with every single step you take, as you step down to the eighth step. Notice how your perspective may be changing around you as you descend lower and lower down the stairs, moving down to the seventh stair. Now, step down to the sixth stair. When you are ready, step again down to the fifth stair, feeling your relaxation doubling once again as you sink deeper and deeper into a state of relaxation and calmness. Now, step down to the fourth stair. As you look before you, you can see a chair coming into your view when you step down again to the third stair. As you step down to the second stair, you can see that the chair looks incredibly comfy, and you cannot wait to go feel your relaxation triple when you sit in it as you step down to the first stair and then off the stairs.

When you get off the stairs at the bottom, see yourself walking up to that chair and sitting in it. Notice that this chair is the comfiest chair you have ever sat in, and upon sitting in it, you feel your entire state relaxing ten times deeper as you sink into the chair. Feel yourself becoming so calm that you are able to simply fade away in this space.

As you sit there, notice your awareness turning inward into your body. As your awareness turns inward, draw your focus down into your fat cells. See each cell sitting there, hugging your body, and keeping you warm and comfortable in your current state. Notice how each cell feels confident that it is serving a purpose, and sits proudly in its position. As you look at each of these fat cells, realize that they are not there to cause you harm or destruction, but because they genuinely believe they are meant to be there. They believe they are serving an important job for you and your life.

As you draw your awareness even closer into these cells, I want you to pick one up in your hand. See this small round cell sitting in your hand, proudly serving a purpose in your life. As you hold it, thank the cell for all that it has done, and with complete gratitude, let it know that you no longer need it to help you anymore. Cup the cell between your hands and feel it shrinking all the way down until it vanishes between your palms.

Again, pick up another cell and hold it in your hands. With deep gratitude in your heart, thank it for serving its purpose and let it know that you no longer need its help. Wish it well as you cup it between your palms and shrink it all the way down until it vanishes.

Keep doing this with your fat cells as you continue to pick them up, express gratitude for their service, and then shrink them down in your palms until they vanish completely. One by one, let each fat cell know that it is no longer needed and that you are grateful for all that it has provided you with until this point in your life. Let your remaining cells know that you now require less fat in your body so that you can restore your health and start to feel better and better.

As you get to the end of the fat cells, notice that you look around and no fat cells remain. All you see are healthy cells that support important functions in your body like cell regrowth, digestion, and circulation. Express deep gratitude for every single cell in your body and the work it is doing, and allow yourself to release this perspective as you draw your awareness back into your body. See your awareness growing beyond the size of your small cells and back into the awareness of yourself as you come back into the room where you presently sit. Feel yourself awakening from your meditation now, as you open your eyes and feel different within your body.

From now on, when you go through your daily life, notice how even though some of your fat cells continue to remain, you can almost see them disappearing. Continue to express gratitude for each cell and all that it has done to attempt to support your survival, and allow it to peacefully fade away as you allow yourself to come back into a state of lean health.

A Deep Meditation for Weight Loss

This is a one-hour meditation that is going to help you achieve weight loss in your life. You should do this meditation once a week at first, and then once every two weeks as you start to notice more lasting changes in your lifestyle and behavior. This meditation will take you much deeper than the simple daily weight loss meditation or fat-burning meditation. For that reason, you are likely going to see far more significant mental and behavioral changes following your session.

This particular meditation should not be done while you are falling asleep, as you do want to stay alert and active throughout it to the best of your ability. While it is okay if you fall asleep while listening to it, you should not encourage yourself to fall asleep as you do want to allow your conscious mind to observe the changes you are making with this meditation. With that being said, you are going to want to relax deeply so that your conscious mind does not attempt to take over control. For that reason, you should lie down in a comfortable position with a pillow and a light blanket in an uninterrupted area as you engage in this deep meditation for weight loss.

The Meditation

We are going to start this meditation by doing a deep relaxation breathing method that will help you completely relax into the moment. I want you to start by laying down in a comfortable position and elongating your spine to open up your airways. You can also sit with a tall spine if you have a comfortable chair to sit in for this. With your chest nice and open, I want you to begin to draw your focus to your breath. Listen to and feel the gentle current of your breath coming in, circulating through your lungs, and being released back into the air around you. Feel yourself completely relaxing into your natural breath as you allow yourself to begin to slow down your breath, creating space for you to relax completely. Breathe in as slowly as you can, feeling your chest and stomach rise as you fill your lungs and diaphragm with air. Then, breathe out slowly, feeling your chest and stomach fall as you let the air from your lungs and diaphragm escape gently. Continue breathing gently as you allow yourself to relax deeper and deeper with each breath, feeling the current growing calmer and more relaxing each time you inhale and exhale.

I want you just to sit in this space for a few moments, meditating with your breath and feeling the entirety of your presence. Feel yourself relaxing completely as you allow yourself to sink deeper and deeper into the here and now, and let everything else that is going on around you simply fade away. If you hear any noises around you, focus on them for a moment, and then let them fade away as you draw your awareness back to your breath. If you notice something that draws your attention away, give it a moment of mindfulness before letting it fade away as you come back to your breath.

Continue letting yourself come back to your breath over and over as you sink deeper into this moment.

When your mind begins to feel completely relaxed, I want you to focus on bringing your body deeper into this state of calmness. Visualize a warm golden light washing through your feet, erasing any stress you may be carrying as your feet relax completely. With each breath in and out, feel this warm light drawing higher and higher up your body, relaxing you even deeper. Feel it washing through your ankles, your shins, your knees, and your thighs. Feel this warm light drawing through your glutes, hips, and pelvis as you continue to breathe in and out. When you are ready, draw this warm golden light in through your abdomen, stomach, and lower back. Let it rise higher into your chest, upper back, and shoulders. Feel your entire torso relaxing as you continue to allow this golden light to circulate through your body and release any stress that you may be carrying within you. As you breathe in again, feel the golden light moving down your shoulders, through your biceps and elbows, and into your forearms and wrists. Feel it circulating in your hands and fingers, all the way down to your fingertips as you completely relax your shoulders, arms, and hands. Breathe in again, letting this warm golden light move up into your neck, scalp, and face as you breathe out and feel everything relaxing completely within you.

Allow yourself to meditate in this space for several moments, feeling the energy of relaxation sinking deeper with each breath. The more you breathe, the more relaxed you feel. The more relaxed you feel, the more present you become, and the easier it is for you to connect to this moment and to your heart. As you connect to your heart, you can feel yourself connecting into your heart's desire, which is to be a healthier, stronger, more vivacious, and happier version of yourself.

Draw on the energy of that desire now, as you allow it to rise up to the surface and come into your space of awareness now. Visualize yourself at your healthiest. See what your body looks like, feels like, and moves like. See how easy it is for you to engage in the things that matter to you when you are healthier because your body gives you the flexibility, freedom, and energy that you need to do the things that you care most about. Spend a few moments creating an image in your mind of something you might be doing when you are living as your healthiest, strongest, and happiest version of yourself. Begin lacing that image with details of who you are and what you are doing, and putting together other details that are relevant to you and your healthier self.

Where are you? What does that place look like, sound like, smell like, and feel like? What are you doing there, and how does it feel to be doing that? See if you can visualize yourself touching or interacting with something in this space. Maybe you are walking, holding your dog's leash, or hugging someone that you care about. Perhaps you are hiking, and you can feel fresh air moving through your lungs, or you are laughing and enjoying good company, and you notice that it truly feels amazing to be you. Let yourself interact with this image for several moments as you continue to breathe in and out, relaxing in this space. Keep your eyes closed, and keep yourself as relaxed as you can in this space.

As you continue breathing, imagine that each breath you are taking is the breath of your future, healthier, slimmer self. Feel how easy and fluid those breaths move in and out of your body, and notice how comfortable it feels to breathe from your healthier body. Connect to your future self through this breath more and more as you inhale and relax and exhale and relax. Notice how good you feel and how proud you feel about being in this new space with your new body. If you desire, you may want to run your hands down your body and feel how slim and fit you feel. Spend time getting to know your body, possibly even looking at it in a mirror where you can admire all of the work you have put in, and the health that you have received out of it. Although you may be excited, overjoyed, or incredibly happy, notice that you also carry a certain mindfulness with you. A mindfulness of where you came from, and the work you put into having this health that your heart desired. Feel connected to that mindfulness and that state of comfort that you have within your new body and your new life.

Now, draw your focus to your heart. Feel your heart beating. Notice that with every single breath, you are drawing closer and closer to that future, healthier, slimmer version of yourself. Feel each heartbeat bringing that vivacious version of you forward and locking it into your body more and more as you continue to effortlessly lose the weight that you have been carrying and wishing to release for so long. Notice that with each breath and each heartbeat, losing weight becomes easier and easier. You find yourself effortlessly shedding pounds as you carve your healthier, leaner, stronger body out of your current self. Feel grateful knowing that you are coming closer and closer to having the body and health that you desire.

When you are ready, release this image of yourself and begin to become aware of your current body. Feel yourself awakening back into the room. Notice how connected you feel to the present moment, as you gently shake out your legs and arms, encouraging them to wake up and return to the present moment. Then, open your eyes and bring yourself fully back into the present moment. As you go about your day to day routines, remember that you have locked this truth of effortless weight loss into your awareness, heart, and subconscious mind. Feel yourself having an easier and easier time losing weight and returning to your best state of health each time your heartbeats, and each time you take a breath. Trust that you are losing weight and that you can effortlessly follow this weight loss plan to help you achieve the body that you desire most out of your life.

Meditation for Cutting Calories

This meditation is an excellent meditation to help you cut calories, allowing you to decrease the amount of food that you are eating on a daily basis. This is a 10-15-minute meditation that will support you in reducing cravings while also reducing your food intake on a daily basis. The goal of this particular meditation is to reduce calorie intake without causing you to starve yourself, so the goal will ultimately be to help you choose healthier meals that help you feel fuller longer, while also cutting out unnecessary snacking in between meals.

You should engage in this meditation at the beginning of the day, or any time you feel yourself experiencing difficulty with food cravings or moderation. That way, you can encourage yourself to stay on track with your weight loss goals. With that being said, you should make sure that you are sitting up with a straight spine during this particular meditation so that you stay engaged and do not lose your energy or motivation following this particular meditation.

The Meditation

Start this meditation by sitting upright in a comfortable position with your spine long and tall and your awareness soft and gentle. When you are ready, I want you to begin to draw your awareness into the center of your chest, directly behind your sternum. As you do, notice how it rises and falls with each breath you take. As you breathe in, feel your sternum pushing away from your spine, and as you breathe out, feel it falling back toward your spine. Continue to focus on this space for four breaths as you relax into this position and enjoy your meditation.

When you start to feel yourself relaxing, I want you to start visualizing yourself, putting together a meal for yourself. Start with breakfast. See yourself filling your plate with healthy options that fill you up without wasting calories. Notice how easy it is to fill your plate with things that are healthy for you, and that helps you feel your best. Allow yourself to begin feeling excited about the food options on that plate, noticing that you are genuinely craving them and looking forward to this meal. Visualize yourself taking a bite of the food, and imagine how amazing it tastes. Notice how you feel yourself being completely satisfied by this food and that you do not have any reason to snack on anything in between because you are so content with your meal.

When it does come time to have a snack, or your next meal, see yourself having the desire to indulge in something healthy again. Notice how easy it is for you to pass up on junk foods or foods that do not support your health because you genuinely enjoy eating things that are healthier for you. See yourself easily opting for healthier food choices, and enjoying each food option that you choose. Feel how great it is that being healthy, cutting calories, and losing weight can be so *delicious*.

Now, when you are ready, bring your awareness back into your present body. Feel yourself awakening into your body, coming back into your conscious state of awareness. Then, when you are ready, you can go about your day once again. Feel yourself effortlessly gravitating toward healthier meal options all day as you focus more on what is going to help you feel healthy, satisfied, and fulfilled from your meals.

Strategies and Mind Exercises for Cutting Calories

In addition to using hypnosis itself, you can also use specific strategies and mind exercises that can help you cut calories and burn fat faster. These six strategies and mindset exercises can help you reinforce the changes you are creating through your daily hypnosis sessions. This way, you are more likely to stay on track longer and increase the amount of time you experience between regression periods.

Affirmations

Affirmations can be an incredible way to keep your mindset focused on healthy. When you are working on changing your subconscious mind, repeating affirmations to yourself can help reinforce the changes you are making during meditations. Affirmations, then, allow you to empower yourself to believe in these changes and continue to adhere to them as you go along in life. Some people will use just one or two affirmations, whereas others will have multiple affirmations that they use depending on what situation they are presently in. In Chapter 4, you can find 300 affirmations to help you cut calories and lose weight faster.

Eating with the Right Mindset

When you set aside time to eat during the day, make sure that you are eating with the right mindset. You want to be eating from a place of being genuinely hungry, and you want to eat with the mindset of wanting to nourish your body. If you find yourself eating from the mindset of desperation, cravings, or overwhelming emotions, you will likely find yourself eating foods that are less than healthy for you. You should always take a few moments to ask yourself: "why am I eating?" and "what am I choosing to nourish my body with?" Your answers should be: because I am genuinely hungry and with something nutritious.

Short Meditations

Meditations are a great way to help keep you on track with your healthy eating. In this particular chapter, we discussed three great shorter meditations that you can use to help you eat healthier on a day to day basis. Short meditations are great because they allow you the opportunity to quickly get your mindset back on track and keep yourself focused. They can easily be used in a short period of time to keep yourself focused and eating healthier while supporting your weight loss goals.

Eating Foods, You Enjoy

If you are trying to lose weight through a diet that you genuinely do not enjoy, you are going to have a hard time sticking to it. Food is something that has the capacity to give us joy and actually stimulates our reward center in our brain. This means that every time you eat something you enjoy; you genuinely derive pleasure from it and feel your best. Eating a diet that you do not enjoy essentially robs you of that pleasure, meaning you will be more likely to choose food options that are not great for you. As you work on weight loss, make sure that you are eating healthier foods that you genuinely enjoy so that you are more likely to reach for them over anything else.

Making Eating an Experience

As you eat, make sure that you make eating an experience. Slow down, indulge in each bite, and strive to taste every single bite you have. Chew thoroughly, and allow yourself to feel completely satisfied with everything you eat. Making eating about the experience rather than about the chore of feeding yourself means that you are more likely to gain pleasure and joy out of what you are eating in the first place. As well, you are more likely to focus on eating only when you are hungry, rather than eating to fill the time or eating because you are feeling emotional.

Mindful Eating

Lastly, engage in mindful eating. When you are using hypnosis and meditation as a way to support you in weight loss, mindful eating is a great practice that goes hand in hand with that. You can help yourself lose weight by intuitively picking your meals and practicing portion control. Rather than letting yourself indulge in habits or in the cravings of your body, let yourself mindfully decide what is the best meal option for you, and what portion you should be eating. Notice when you are full and stop eating, and notice when you are hungry and opt for something nutritious. If you notice you have a craving for a certain treat, indulge in a small portion of it to satisfy your craving, rather than strictly denying yourself from it. Following these mindful patterns mean that you will be more likely to stay on track with your weight loss goals, rather than trying to force yourself to stick to habits or eating behaviors that do not feel right for you.

Chapter 3: Portion Control Hypnosis

Portion control tends to be a skill that many people struggle with. Knowing how to eat just enough to help yourself feel satisfied and full, without overeating, can be challenging. This is made even more challenging if you tend to be a stress eater or someone who goes long periods of time without eating and then binge eats. Portion control is an incredibly important element of weight loss as it provides you with the opportunity to get the proper nutrients into your body without overdoing it. As well, if you choose to satisfy one of your cravings or enjoy something more indulgent, portion control enables you to do so without going overboard.

The truth is: most people can eat anything in moderation and not suffer any unwanted consequences from eating that food. For example, if you want to enjoy a piece of brownie with your coffee at the café because you have been craving a brownie, there is typically nothing wrong with doing that. The key is to make sure that you enjoy the brownie, and then you *stop.* Rather than enjoying that brownie, then eating another piece, then going home and having even more junk food, enjoy that one brownie and then let yourself get back on track with healthy eating. When you can mindfully engage in portion control this way, you can eat just about anything you want without having any problems.

In fact, many famous diets rely more on portion control than anything else because they recognize that portion control is more effective than restricting what people can and cannot eat. The key with portion control is knowing how to actually feel satisfied by your controlled portions, and knowing how to stay committed to them. For many people, this can be challenging. You may feel so happy about eating your brownie or your piece of cake that you want more immediately after. Of course, if you immediately indulge, then you are not effectively engaging in portion control. However, if you instead let yourself enjoy that piece as much as you possibly can and then go back to eating healthy immediately after, then there was no big deal.

Rather than relying solely on portion control as a tool, it is important that you rewire your mind around why you struggle with portion control as it is. Getting to the root cause of your own struggles with portion control, healing your overeating challenges, and rewiring your mind around portion control can be incredibly helpful in allowing you to get what you need out of your diet. This way, rather than dealing with that internal conflict around, "I should stop," you stop naturally because your mind is already wired to stop naturally. As you might suspect, this can be done with subconscious work and hypnosis. However, there are also some conscious-level changes that you should make and things you should become mindful of so that you can navigate portion control both with your conscious mind and your new subconscious habits. This way, you are more likely to be successful with portion control in general.

Why Do People Overeat?

There are many different reasons why people overeat, although emotions and poor eating habits tend to be the most common ones that people experience. Another reason behind overeating can actually be an eating disorder, which may be caused by underlying conditions such as depression or anxiety, genetics, or other illnesses. If you do have an issue with compulsive overeating and struggle to keep it under control, talking to your doctor is an important way of ruling out possible illness factors that could be contributing to your problems.

When it comes to emotions, everything from stress and anxiety to sadness or discomfort can trigger someone to want to overeat. Believe it or not, the majority of our serotonin and other hormones are produced in the gut. Because of this, when you are feeling stressed out, anxious, sad, or otherwise uncomfortable, you might find yourself craving food. Most people will find themselves craving something specific, such as sweet or salty foods. Other people may find that they are willing to eat whatever is nearby in order to receive that "release" from having something yummy to eat. While overeating due to emotional causes every once in a while, may not necessarily be a bad thing, it is easy for this behavior to turn into a habit. Many people find themselves struggling with overeating due to emotional causes, although stress and sadness tend to be the leading causes of overeating.

Poor eating habits can also contribute to overeating. If you find yourself skipping breakfast or lunch on a regular basis, you may find yourself overcompensating at dinner time because you are so hungry. Learning how to fix your eating habits by eating more consistently and eating healthier portions at proper meal times is an important way to take care of yourself. Eating regular meals will prevent you from binge eating later on due to being excessively hungry.

Getting to the Root Cause of Your Binge Eating

Understanding your own binge eating habits is important, as this allows you to develop a conscious awareness and a sense of mindfulness around why you are binge eating in the first place. When you are able to understand why you binge eat, resolving the root cause of your binge eating becomes easier because you know what to look for and what to be aware of. Getting to the root cause of your own binge eating can be done by reflecting on your own binge eating cycles and, if necessary, tracking your binge eating cycles so that you can start to identify any possible patterns that exist around your binge eating behaviors. You can easily do this by keeping a food diary, which is a journal where you log everything you have eaten in a day. Make sure that you write down the time that you ate, what you ate, and how much you ate. Track everything, including little snacks in between. They may not seem significant, but you might be surprised to see how they add up and what comes of those snacks. Often, people find that they are unaware of how problematic their snacking has actually become until they begin to track it.

As you begin looking for the root cause of your binge eating, you might find that there are actually a few root causes. Often, however, most binge eating patterns can be traced back to one "major" root problem that seems to create more problems than the rest. For example, you might find that you have poor eating habits and often find yourself craving low-quality food, but you might realize that this largely stems from you being an emotional eater. Or, you might find that you are an emotional eater because you have poor eating problems and so you realize that, during a moment of stress, eating is one thing you can take care of while everything else might seem out of your control.

It is important that you take the time to identify every single root cause of your binge eating and not just the one that stands out the most. If you are going to have the biggest impact on changing your binge eating patterns, you are going to need to know everything that contributes to your binge eating so that you can be mindful of what might be triggering this behavior. If you do not focus on and heal *all* of your root causes for binge eating, you might find yourself binge eating out of habit and justifying it by different root causes every single time. The more thorough you can be with healing this, the more effective you will be, too.

With that being said, you may find it to be particularly overwhelming to attempt to actually resolve all of your root causes at once, especially if you have a few. If it does feel overwhelming, you can focus instead on just dealing with the biggest one and then healing one root cause at a time. This way, you can make a significant impact on healing your binge eating problems, but you are still able to remain mindful and aware of your other binge eating triggers.

Learning to Avoid Temptations and Triggers

Once you have a clear understanding of what your binge eating cycles and patterns are like, you can start implementing change to help you avoid temptations and triggers. There are many ways that you can reasonably avoid temptations and triggers when it comes to eliminating binge eating; however, you are going to need to focus just as much on your mindset as you do on your behaviors if you want to truly change. This is where meditation is going to help you really begin to start engaging in proper portion control so that you are no longer at risk of binge eating anymore. With meditation and hypnosis, you can begin to resolve the deep subconscious reasons behind your binge eating behaviors so that you have an easier time actually adhering to your changes. The more you engage in this deep healing, the easier it is going to be for you to make conscious and mindful changes in your eating habits, too.

As you use meditation and hypnosis to help you stop binge eating, you also need to focus on actually intentionally avoiding temptations and triggers. There are many practical ways that you can mindfully eliminate these temptations and triggers from your life. For example, you might intentionally stop buying the types of foods that you regularly binge eat so that the temptation no longer exists to begin with. You might also make sure that you eat on a consistent schedule so that you are no longer fasting to the point of being so hungry that you cannot stop yourself. If that is hard for you, picking up habits like meal prepping is a great opportunity for you to prevent yourself from waiting too long between meals and then binge eating as a way to make up for missing out on foods.

Another important way to start overcoming binge eating is to recognize that emotions can be a major trigger. In recognizing that, you can choose to identify and enlist new coping methods to help you navigate emotions in a healthier way that does not include binge eating. This way, you are more likely to manage your emotions with proper emotional management tools, rather than trying to numb yourself with the satisfaction that you get from snacking on junk foods.

If you find that anything else not listed here tends to be a temptation or trigger for you to binge eat, make sure that you remain aware of it and that you start offsetting it by changing your habits and behaviors. The more you can become aware of your own patterns and cycles, the easier it will be for you to find ways to overcome these patterns and cycles so that you can have a healthier relationship with food.

Tips for Managing Stress to Avoid Emotional Eating

No matter what your binge eating cycles are like, stress is almost sure to encourage you to engage in emotional eating. When it comes to stress and its ability to influence your dietary behaviors, there are generally two ways that it can happen. The first is that you find yourself feeling stressed out, and you binge eat as a way to create some form of comfort in your life so that you are not feeling quite as stressed out anymore. The other way includes you feeling so stressed out that you feel that you cannot eat, and then binge eating when your body cannot take the stress-induced fasting any longer. In either scenario, stress can negatively affect your diet, and can also turn into a negative coping method that worsens your binge eating in the future, too. Furthermore, both of these behavioral patterns around stress and eating can lead to weight gain, which means that they are not productive to your goals of weight *loss*.

Managing stress to avoid emotional eating largely revolves around you learning how to properly cope with and manage your stress. The more proactive you can be in dealing with your stress, the less likely you are to seek out behaviors like binge eating as an opportunity to help you overcome the stress that you are experiencing. People who routinely experience problematic binge eating due to stress or other emotions will often turn to healthier practices such as meditating, preventative self-care, and routine relaxation practices to help them reduce stress. This way, they are less likely to engage in emotional eating in the first place.

When it comes to dealing with bursts of higher stress levels, meditating can be incredibly helpful in assisting you with bringing your stress levels back down. Meditations like the chakra meditation we do in chapter 5 can work wonders in helping you lower your overall stress. This way, you are more likely to feel at peace and less likely to feel the need to deal with your stress through less healthy means, such as through overeating.

Preventative self-care measures that can help you deal with your stress are incredibly useful in warding off stress in the first place. For example, budgeting more effectively so that you are not so worried about money, creating a savings account, exercising on a regular basis, and spending time with loved ones are all great ways to avoid scenarios where your stress may rise unnecessarily. The more effective you are at dealing with areas of your life that typically result in stress, the more effective you will be in eliminating your stress. Or, when it cannot be completely eliminated, at least minimizing it so that you can feel more at peace in your life.

Routine relaxation practices are similar to preventative self-care, except that they are more focused on day to day practices that are meant to help you relax no matter what has triggered your stress. For example, some people come home after work every day and enjoy some time gardening, reading a book, or simply resting on the couch with their eyes closed so that they have time to decompress from the day they have had. Other people like to take a candlelit bath, go for a walk, or even play a game on their laptop as a way to destress. The idea here is that you find a healthy way to decompress each time you feel stressed and that you do it on a daily basis so that your stress does not begin to rise too much in the first place.

When it comes to managing your stress to avoid overeating, the best thing you can do is continue to try out new routines and rituals until you find practices that help you destress without overeating. The exact "formula" for destressing will be different for everyone, so you are going to have to take some time to find that information out for yourself. The better you understand your own needs around stress and how to relax, the more likely you are to be able to come up with a practice that is actually going to help you destress in the first place.

Learning to Eat Intuitively

Eating intuitively and using hypnosis for weight loss go hand in hand. Intuitive eating is a practice where you take the time to actually get to know your body and start to understand your own personal eating cues. In doing so, you increase your awareness around what your body actually wants, when, and how much. It can take some time to learn how to intuitively eat, particularly if you have been significantly disconnected from your own intuition for quite some time. Your intuition is often also referred to as your "gut feeling" and it gives you information about how you are doing and what you need or want more of in your life. This includes nutrition and exercise.

Intuitive eating can be accomplished by first taking the time to get to know your body's cues around hunger. Spend time getting to know what it feels like when you are hungry and thirsty. Get to know what it feels like when you start getting *too* hungry so that you are less likely to ignore your hunger pangs for such a long period of time, to the point where you end up binge eating to make up for your hunger period. In addition to knowing what it feels like to be hungry and too hungry, get to know what it feels like to be full. Many people do not realize that being full is more of a feeling of being satisfied than a feeling of physically being full, which is why many people eat to the point where they feel "stuffed." Feeling "stuffed" means that you have eaten too much. You should always feel satisfied and comfortable after eating a proper sized meal, not nauseous, or like you overdid it.

As you get to know your hunger cues, also start to understand your cravings. Most of us find that we start craving or thinking about a certain food or a certain flavor around the same time that we get hungry. These are great indicators as to what we need in our diet and what our body is asking for. If you have not been eating healthy in the past, you might find that your cravings often lean toward sugar, chocolate, fatty foods, and other junk foods. This is because, until now, you have trained your body to see these as the food sources to look out for. Often, this happens as a result of binge eating because you either wait too long to eat then fill up on "fast fuel" like sugar, or you eat to soothe yourself, so you fill up on sugars that help boost your "feel good" hormones inside of your body and your brain.

A great way to heal these cravings is to recognize that when you are craving junk food, you are often not actually craving junk food but instead the type of energy or nutrient that this particular junk food offers you. For example, if you are craving chocolate, you are likely in need of more magnesium in your diet. You can acquire healthy sources of magnesium through fruits, vegetables, seeds, and nuts. Or, if you are craving sugary foods, you may need more chromium, carbon, phosphorus, sulfur, or tryptophan in your diet. Eating broccoli, grapes, cheese, chicken, fresh fruits, chicken, beef, fatty fish, eggs, dairy, nuts, veggies, grains, cranberries, horseradish, cabbage, cauliflower, cheese, raisins, sweet potatoes, or spinach would be a healthier alternative. This way, you get what your body is craving without relying on an unhealthy food source to get it. If you are craving bread, pasta, and other simple carbs, you might be in need of more nitrogen in your diet. Nitrogen can be acquired through high protein foods like meat, fatty fish, nuts, beans, and chia seeds. If you are craving oily foods, you may be lacking calcium, which can be acquired through organic milk, cheese, and green leafy vegetables. Lastly, if you are craving salty foods, it is likely that you need chloride or silicon in your diet, which can be acquired through fatty fish, goats' milk, cashews, and other nuts and seeds.

Learning how to understand what your body actually wants and needs and giving it that is the best way to make sure that you are taking proper care of your body. You will likely find that over time, your body begins to intuitively crave the healthier alternatives over the junkier foods because it begins to realize that these foods offer far more nutrition and do far less damage to your body. As a result, you will find that your cravings naturally subside and your body heals from the damage that may have been caused by these less healthy nutritional sources and eating behaviors.

It is important to understand that eating intuitively is, in most cases, the only way to eat in a way that is actually going to satisfy your needs while also helping you lose weight safely. Unlike dieting, intuitive eating does not discriminate against what you can and cannot eat but instead encourages you to work together with your body to improve your overall health. In most cases, you can still safely eat a sugary dessert or a piece of chocolate from time to time, as long as you are following your intuition, and you are not overdoing it. If you do find that you are overdoing it, chances are you are eating based on emotions or habit, and not based on what your intuition is actually guiding you to do.

Getting Support When You Need It

Getting the right diet can be incredibly challenging, especially if you have had problems with your diet in the past. If you have struggled with binge eating or junk food cravings in the past, or if you have struggled with yo-yo dieting or poor body image issues, taking care of yourself through your diet can be incredibly challenging. You might find that no matter how much you know about eating healthy and taking care of yourself, you find it to be incredibly challenging to implement your knowledge into your everyday life. This is because, no matter how much you know, emotions, and habits can be strong and powerful and can be incredibly difficult for you to break.

In some cases, you may not be able to break your own habits or emotional connections to eating without getting help. If you find that you are struggling and that, despite how much knowledge you have around eating healthy, you are still binge eating or unable to control yourself, getting help can be invaluable. Help can be anything from an accountability buddy to a counselor or a weight loss group that you join to help you get and stay on track with your weight loss goals.

If you are seeking out an accountability buddy, a trusted family member or friend can be incredibly helpful and can go a long way. Make sure to choose someone that you feel comfortable talking to, that you will be honest with, and that will not enable you to stray away from your goals. You want someone who is going to listen compassionately and be firm in guiding you forward and motivating you to stay on track so that you are more likely to stay committed to your weight loss goals. As well, this should be someone that you can feel confident is going to be gentle when you are having a hard time, as in some cases having an accountability buddy that pushes you too hard can lead to you feeling overwhelmed or even more stressed. Naturally, if you are struggling with stress eating, this can make your wellbeing a lot more difficult for you to manage.

If you have been dealing with a fair bit of stress or emotions that are triggering you to binge eat, having a counselor to help you through your weight loss journey can be incredibly helpful. Counselors can help you dig into the root causes of your binge eating or your poor eating habits. They can also support you with creating healthier ways for coping with stress and other challenging emotions so that you are less likely to turn to and rely on binge eating to help you deal with troubling emotions. This way, you will be more likely to use healthier coping methods that actually help you dig into the root cause of your emotions and heal them, rather than numbing them out with things like food.

Weight loss groups can be helpful, too. Within weight loss groups, you can find support from other people who are also seeking to lose weight. You also tend to have a group "leader" who can guide you and help keep you on track with your goals. Many people find that having a group of people to embrace the journey with is helpful because you stop feeling so alone with your troubles, and you have more people to help keep you accountable. This way, if you find yourself struggling, you have more people to rely on to help motivate you to keep going. Likewise, groups often have weigh-ins and other accountable practices that help motivate you to stay on track.

When it comes to getting help, you need to take the route that works best for you. If you would prefer to just have an accountability partner, or just have a counselor, or just have a weight loss group to help you, then go with that. If you would rather have a mixture of two or even all three of these support measures to help you keep going, then create a mixed support team. The key here is to make sure that you feel supported in the choices that you make, and to make sure that you feel confident that you have someone to fall back on any time you are struggling. Whether that is just one person or many people, does not matter so much as how willing you are to lean on your support team and actually allow them to help you stay motivated to keep going.

Forgiving Yourself for Your Dietary Mistakes

Forgiveness is an underrated and extremely important element of weight loss. Often times, people who are in the position of wanting or needing to lose weight fail to acknowledge the fact that they have been feeling incredibly frustrated with themselves. Anger, frustration, disappointment, and sadness directed at yourself when you are on this journey are all incredibly normal feelings to have. They can also be painful and overwhelming if you do not take the time to acknowledge them, forgive yourself, and heal them as you experience them.

You may find yourself feeling angry, frustrated, disappointed, or sad that you let yourself gain so much weight. You may fail to acknowledge the fact that it was not intentional, or that it had causes that were beyond your control, especially if your weight gain was related to medical conditions or a lack of education around healthy eating. Regardless of what lead to you gaining weight, you may feel contempt for yourself for "allowing" it to happen, and that may make it difficult for you to truly commit to losing weight. When you sit in anger and frustration with yourself, it can be difficult to accept yourself as you are now and work toward improving your wellbeing through weight loss. Forgiving yourself for not knowing better or for not doing better, or even forgiving yourself for blaming yourself for something that was beyond your control, is important. The more you can forgive yourself, the more likely you are to acknowledge that your weight is something you want to work on. Through that, you will be able to work on weight loss from a *peaceful* frame of mind.

Studies have shown that those who accept themselves as they are and forgive their mistakes are more likely to lose the excess weight and keep it off than those who refuse to forgive themselves. Refusing to forgive yourself can create a massive amount of stress inside of you that makes it difficult for you to stay focused on exercising, eating healthy, and improving your wellness. Many people find that this difficulty in forgiving themselves worsens their self-esteem and self-confidence, which keeps them in the unhealthy cycle of behaviors and patterns that lead to their weight gain in the first place. If you want to overcome these cycles, you need to be willing to forgive yourself for your past choices, mistakes, and experiences that may or may not have been beyond your control.

Another area where you need to master forgiveness is in the process of change. As you move away from old habits and behaviors and into a new way of looking after your body, you are all but guaranteed to make mistakes. You are going to have days or even weeks where you fall back into old patterns. Some people even fall back into old patterns and stay trapped in them for *years.* This happens because they are unwilling to forgive themselves for making a mistake, and so they fall back into the cycle of contempt and low self-esteem and self-worth.

If you want to be able to continue moving forward with your wellness and to jump back on track as quickly as possible, you need to be willing to forgive yourself for any mistakes you make. This means anytime you overeat, engage in an old eating pattern, opt for an unhealthy food choice, or otherwise make a "mistake" in your diet, you forgive yourself. Upon forgiving yourself, make sure that you also commit to taking that experience into account so that you can make better choices. Make an honest effort to do better next time so that each time you forgive yourself, you give yourself a reason to believe that your commitment to yourself genuinely means something. When you can forgive yourself and believe that your commitment to bettering yourself and your life means something, you begin to build your self-esteem. Through that, things like portion control begin to become easier, and you find yourself naturally gravitating toward taking better care of yourself.

Meditation for Portion Control

The following is a simple 5-10-minute meditation that you can do before you sit down to eat a meal. Using it is going to help you intentionally engage in portion control so that you can refrain from overeating. You should use this meditation in conjunction with other practices from this chapter so that you are more likely to experience a healthy approach to portion control. Adding this meditation into the mixture will ensure that you are approaching your improved portion control from a deep subconscious level, allowing you to experience even more success in committing to moderation and healing your body through weight loss.

When you do this meditation, you should be actively sitting up with a straight spine. Laying down may lead to you feeling too tired or creating excess calmness in your day, which may lead to you struggling to maintain energy throughout the day.

The Meditation

I want you to begin by intentionally taking one nice deep breath into your belly, pressing your belly button and chest forward with your breath. Then, when you breathe out, let your belly button and chest drawback toward your spine. Feel the movement of your body as it naturally flows with each breath. Do not try to control the rate at which you breathe or the speed at which you breathe, but instead focus on how your body naturally breathes in and out for you. Feel your body intuitively drawing in and circulating oxygen throughout your body, and exhaling carbon dioxide from your body just as easily. Notice how calm your body feels with each breath. Feel how breathing is so natural, so simple, so basic, and yet continues to be one of the strongest stress relievers we have. Meditate here with your breath for a few moments as you sink deeply into this feeling of trusting your body and your intuition to take care of you through each breath.

Now, I want you to draw your awareness even deeper, into your stomach. Pause for a moment and notice any hunger that may be arising within your body. Take into account what this hunger feels like, and what cues your body is giving you that indicates that it is time to eat. Feel yourself acknowledging and becoming aware of your own needs and trusting that your intuition is giving you the right information about your body.

As you start listening to your intuition about your hunger, ask yourself: "How hungry am I?" pay attention to the answer that rises. Are you hungry for a snack or a full meal? Be mindful of how much fod your body genuinely wants and how much it needs.

Now, ask yourself, "what am I truly hungry for?" and pay close attention. Trust that whatever answer comes in is correct, and be willing to work together with your body to find the best source of nutrition for you and your wellbeing. Trust that once you are done this meditation, you can opt for something healthier and more nutritious that will help your body meet its needs.

As you continue to sit with your intuition, develop a trust in your inner knowingness and your inner ability to recognize your hunger cues. Ask your body to be honest about when you feel full, and ask it to help you naturally stop craving food so that you can stop eating when your body feels full. Affirm that you want to take care of your body and earn its trust by serving it in the way that it truly needs to be served. Affirm that you are worthy of deeply enjoying healthy portions of food that nourish your body without overwhelming you. Feel yourself being fulfilled and satisfied by these affirmations. Trust that they are true and that your subconscious, unconscious, and conscious mind can all work together to help you manage your eating habits more effectively.

When you are ready to awaken yourself from this meditation, bring your awareness back to your breath, then to your body. Feel yourself gently awakening from this moment of peace, and allow yourself to acknowledge what your body told you it needed. Act on that information and, to the best of your ability, follow your intuition and hunger cues to ensure that you feed yourself an appropriate amount of healthy, nutritious food.

If, during the meditation, your body informed you that it was not actually hungry but instead was in need of emotional support, be sure to avoid emotional eating and instead seek out an alternative way for managing your emotions. The more you can practice following these intuitive cues around emotions and other needs, in addition to your hunger cues, the better you are going to be able to take care of yourself. Through this, you will find yourself naturally engaging in portion control and taking care of your wellbeing through your diet. As a result, you will lose weight faster, easier, and in a healthier manner.

Chapter 4: Affirmation to Cut Calories

Affirmations are a wonderful tool to use alongside hypnosis to help you rewire your brain and improve your weight loss abilities. Affirmations are essentially a tool that you use to remind you of your chosen "rewiring" and to encourage your brain to opt for your newer, healthier mindset over your old unhealthy one. Using affirmations is an important part of anchoring your hypnosis efforts into your daily life, so it is important that you use them on a routine basis.

When using affirmations, it is important that you use ones that are relevant and that are going to actually support you in anchoring your chosen reality into your present reality. In this chapter, we are going to explore exactly what affirmations are and how they work, how to pick ones that are going to work for you, and 300 affirmations that will help set you on your way.

What Are Affirmations, and How Do They Work?

Anytime you repeat something to yourself out loud, or in your thoughts, you are *affirming* something to yourself. We use affirmations on a consistent basis, whether we consciously realize it or not. For example, if you are on your weight loss journey and you repeat "I am never going to lose the weight" to yourself on a regular basis, you are affirming to yourself that you are never going to succeed with weight loss. Likewise, if you are consistently saying, "I will always be fat" or "I am never going to reach my goals" you are affirming those things to yourself, too.

When we use affirmations unintentionally, we often find ourselves using affirmations that can be hurtful and harmful to our psyche and our reality. You might find yourself locking into becoming a mental bully toward yourself as you consistently repeat things to yourself that are unkind and even downright mean. As you do this, you affirm a lower sense of self-confidence, a lack of motivation, and a commitment to a body shape and wellness journey that you do not actually want to maintain.

Affirmations, whether positive or negative, conscious, or unconscious, are always creating or reinforcing the function of your brain and mindset. Each time you repeat something to yourself, your subconscious mind hears it and strives to make it a part of your reality. This is because your subconscious mind is responsible for creating your reality and your sense of identity. It creates both around your affirmations since these are what you perceive as being your absolute truth; therefore, they create a "concrete" foundation for your reality and identity to rest on. If you want to change these two aspects of yourself and your experience, you are going to need to change what you are routinely repeating to yourself so that you are no longer creating a reality and identity rooted in negativity.

In order to change your subconscious experience, you need to consciously choose positive affirmations and repeat them on a constant basis to help you achieve the reality and identity that you truly want. This way, you are more likely to create an experience that reflects what you are looking for, rather than an experience that reflects what your conscious and subconscious mind has automatically picked up on.

The key with affirmations is that you need to understand that your brain does not care if you are creating them on purpose or not. It also does not care if you are creating healthy and positive ones or unhealthy and negative ones. All your subconscious mind cares about is what is repeated to it, and what you perceive as being your absolute truth. It is up to you and your conscious mind to recognize that negative and unhealthy affirmations will hold you back, prevent you from experiencing positive experiences in life, and result in you feeling incapable and unmotivated. Alternatively, consciously choosing healthy and positive affirmations will help you with creating a mindset that is healthier and an identity that actually serves your wellbeing on a mental, physical, emotional, and spiritual level. From there, your responsibility is to consistently repeat these affirmations to yourself until you believe them, and you begin to see them being reflected in your reality.

How Do I Pick and Use Affirmations for Weight Loss?

Choosing affirmations for your weight loss journey requires you to first understand what it is that you are looking for, and what types of positive thoughts are going to help you get there. You can start by identifying what your dream is, what you want your ideal body to look and feel like, and how you want to feel as you achieve your dream of losing weight. Once you have identified what your dream is, you need to identify what current beliefs you have around the dream that you are aspiring to achieve. For example, if you want to lose 25 pounds so that you can have a healthier weight, but you believe that it will be incredibly hard to lose that weight, then you know that your current beliefs are that losing weight is hard. You need to identify every single belief surrounding your weight loss goals and recognize which ones are negative or are limiting and preventing you from achieving your goal of losing weight.

After you have identified which of your beliefs are negative and unhelpful, you can choose affirmations that are going to help you change your beliefs. Typically, you want to choose an affirmation that is going to help you completely change that belief in the opposite direction. For example, if you think "losing weight is hard," your new affirmation could be "I lose the weight effortlessly." Even if you do not believe this new affirmation right now, the goal is to repeat it to yourself enough that it becomes a part of your identity and, inevitably, your reality. This way, you are anchoring in your hypnosis sessions, and you are effectively rewiring your brain in between sessions, too.

As you use affirmations to help you achieve weight loss, I encourage you to do so in a way that is intuitive to your experience. There is no right or wrong way to approach affirmations, as long as you are using them on a regular basis. Once you feel yourself effortlessly believing in an affirmation, you can start incorporating new affirmations into your routine so that you can continue to use your affirmations to improve your wellbeing overall. Ideally, you should always be using positive affirmations even after you have seen the changes you desire, as affirmations are a wonderful way to help naturally maintain your mental, emotional, and physical wellbeing.

What Should I Do with My Affirmations?

After you have chosen what affirmations you want to use, and which ones are going to feel best for you, you need to know what to do with them! The simplest way to use your affirmations is to pick 1-2 affirmations and repeat them to yourself on a regular basis. You can repeat them anytime you feel the need to re-affirm something to yourself, or you can repeat them continually even if they do not seem entirely relevant in the moment. The key is to make sure that you are always repeating them to yourself so that you are more likely to have success in rewiring your brain and achieving the new, healthier, and more effective beliefs that you need to improve the quality of your life.

In addition to repeating your affirmations to yourself, you can also use them in many other ways. One way that people like using affirmations is by writing them down. You can write your affirmations down on little notes and leave them around your house, or you can make a ritual out of writing your affirmations down a certain amount of times per day in a journal so that you are able to routinely work them into your day. Some people will also meditate on their affirmations, meaning that they essentially meditate and then repeat the affirmations to themselves over and over in a meditative state. If repeating your affirmation to yourself like a mantra is too challenging, you can also say your chosen affirmations to yourself on a voice recording track and then repeat them to yourself on loop while you meditate. Other people will create recordings of themselves repeating several affirmations into their voice recorder and then listening to them on loop while they work out, eat, drive to work, or otherwise engage in an activity where affirmations might be useful.

If you really want to make your affirmations effective and get the most out of them, you need to find a way to essentially bombard your brain with this new information. The more effectively you can do this, the more your subconscious brain is going to pick up on it and continue to reinforce your new neural pathways with these new affirmations. Through that, you will find yourself effortlessly and naturally believing in the new affirmations that you have chosen for yourself.

How Are Affirmations Going to Help Me Lose Weight?

Affirmations are going to help you lose weight in a few different ways. First and foremost, and probably most obvious, is the fact that affirmations are going to help you get in the mindset of weight loss. To put it simply: you cannot sit around believing nothing is going to work and expect things to work for you. You need to be able to cultivate a motivated mindset that allows you to create success. If you are unable to believe that it will come true: trust that it will not come true.

As your mindset improves, your subconscious mind is actually going to start changing other things within your body, too. For example, rather than creating desires and cravings for things that are not healthy for you, your body will begin to create desires and cravings for things that are healthy for you. It will also stop creating inner conflict around making the right choices and taking care of yourself. In fact, you may even find yourself actually falling in love with your new diet and your new exercise routine. You will also likely find yourself naturally leaning toward behaviors and habits that are healthier for you without having to try so hard to create those habits. In many cases, you might create habits that are healthy for you without even realizing that you are creating those habits. Rather than having to consciously become aware of the need for habits, and then putting in the work to create them, your body and mind will naturally begin to recognize the need for better habits and will create those habits naturally as well.

Some studies have also suggested that using affirmations will help your brain and subconscious mind actually govern your body differently, too. For example, you may be able to improve your body's ability to digest things and manage your weight naturally by using affirmations and hypnosis. In doing so, you may be able to subconsciously adjust which hormones, chemicals, and enzymes are created within your body to help with things like digestive functions, energy creation, and other weight- and health-related concerns that you may have.

In the next half of this chapter, we are going to explore more than 300 affirmations you can rely on to help you lose your weight, increase your health, and feel better overall. You can use these affirmations as they are, or you can adjust them to match what you need for your own belief system. If you do rewrite them, make sure that you are creating ones that directly reflect what you need to hear so that you can change your beliefs to ones that are more supportive and less limiting.

Affirmations for Self-Control

Self-control is an important discipline to have, and not having it can lead to behaviors that are known for making weight loss more challenging. If you are struggling with self-control, the following affirmations will help you change any beliefs you have around self-control so that you can start approaching food, exercise, weight loss, and wellness in general with healthier beliefs.

1. I have self-control.
2. My willpower is my superpower.
3. I am in complete control of myself in this experience.

4. I make my own choices.

5. I have the power to decide.

6. I am dedicated to achieving my goals.

7. I will make the best choice for me.

8. I succeed because I have self-control.

9. I am capable of working through hardships.

10. I am dedicated to overcoming challenges.

11. My mind is strong, powerful, and disciplined.

12. I am in control of my desires.

13. My mindset is one of success.

14. I become more disciplined every day.

15. Self-discipline comes easily for me.

16. Self-control comes easily for me.

17. I achieve success because I am in control.

18. I find it easier to succeed every day.

19. I see myself as a successful, self-disciplined person.

20. Self-control comes effortlessly for me.

21. Self-control is as natural as breathing.

22. I have control over my thoughts.

23. I have control over my choices.

24. I can trust my willpower to carry me through.

25. I can tap into self-control whenever I need to.

26. My self-control is stronger than my desire.

27. I am incredibly strong with self-control.

28. I easily maintain my self-control in all situations.

29. I see things through to the end.

30. I can depend on myself to make healthy choices.

31. Healthy choices are easy for me to make.

32. It is easy for me to control my impulses.

33. Self-control is my natural state.

34. I will keep going until I reach my goal.

35. I am starting to love the feeling of self-control.

36. I see myself as a successful person.

37. I have unbreakable willpower.

38. I have excellent self-control.

39. I am a highly self-disciplined person.

40. I succeed with every goal I create.

41. I am a highly intentional person.

42. Every day, my self-control gets stronger.

43. I am becoming highly disciplined.

44. I am successful because of my self-discipline.

45. I am a strong, capable person.

46. I am dedicated to achieving my wellness goals.

47. Self-control is one of my greatest strengths.

48. I am in complete control of this situation.

49. I can do this.

50. I am self-aware and capable.

51. I can move forward with self-control and gratitude.

52. I always do what I say I am going to do.

53. I show up as my best self, and I achieve my dreams.

54. I have the willpower to make this happen.

55. I can count on myself to make the right choice.

56. I trust my strength to carry me through.

57. I am becoming stronger every day.

58. I make my choices with self-discipline.

59. I have the discipline to see this through.

60. I make my choices intentionally.

61. I am committed to my success.

Affirmations for Exercise

Exercise is necessary for healthy weight loss, but it can be challenging to commit to. Many people struggle with motivating themselves to exercise, or to exercise enough, to take proper care of their body. If you are struggling with exercising, these affirmations will help motivate you to work out or motivate you to finish your workout on a high note.

1. I am so excited to exercise.
2. I love moving my body.
3. I am focused and ready to exercise.
4. I am showing up at 100%.
5. Today, I will have an excellent workout.
6. I have the courage to see this workout through.
7. My body is becoming stronger every day.
8. I love exercising.
9. Exercising is fun and exciting.
10. I love becoming the best version of myself.
11. Exercising is one of my favorite activities.
12. Exercising makes me feel happy and healthy.
13. I have a strong body and mind.
14. I am confident about my ability to see this through.
15. I can feel myself becoming stronger.
16. I can feel myself becoming leaner.

17. My body is getting healthier every single day.

18. I am transforming my body every day.

19. I am creating the body I have always wanted.

20. Every day I am losing weight.

21. I am getting thinner every single day.

22. Each day I get closer to my ideal weight.

23. I am motivated to take care of my body.

24. I am excited to lose weight in a healthy, natural way.

25. My body is capable of being healthy.

26. I love how flexible my body is becoming.

27. Maintaining my ideal weight is as easy as breathing.

28. My weight is dropping quickly and in a healthy way.

29. I am dedicated to having a stronger body.

30. I feel myself getting stronger every single day.

31. My body deserves a healthy workout.

32. I love creating my dream body.

33. Having a strong body is important to me.

34. I am motivated to reach my fitness goals.

35. I am determined to have a healthier body.

36. I am so proud of myself for my growth.

37. I am strong and motivated.

38. I am committed to having a healthier body.

39. I easily become motivated to exercise.

40. I am capable of having a healthier body.

41. I feel vivacious and healthy.

42. I am in tune with my body.

43. I love how a full workout feels.

44. I feel all of the unhealthy toxins, leaving my body while I work out.

45. Every day I have more stamina.

46. Exercising gets easier and easier.

47. The more I exercise, the better I feel.

48. Exercising helps me sleep better.

49. When I look in the mirror after exercising, I love what I see.

50. I am strong, fit, and capable.

51. Every day I grow closer to my ideal body shape.

52. I exercise with gratitude.

53. I put my all into my workout sessions.

54. Hard work pays off.

55. I take a rest day when I need one.

56. I enjoy working out.

57. I love the burn that affirms my growth.

58. I enjoy participating in exercise.

59. I choose to take proper care of my body.

60. A healthy exercise routine and diet is all I need.

61. Working out helps me feel better.

62. I deserve to feel healthy.

Affirmations for Healthier Habits

Your habits can play a big role in your wellness. From how you eat to how you sleep and how you otherwise take care of yourself, habits are important. As you work toward losing weight and creating a healthier lifestyle, positive affirmations can help you. With the following positive affirmations, you can make committing to your healthier habits much easier.

1. It is easy for me to have healthier habits.
2. I have an easy time eating healthy food.
3. I eat on a regular basis.
4. I choose to eat healthy foods.
5. I move my body on a regular basis.
6. I foster healthy habits, so I can enjoy a healthy body.
7. I always choose the healthy option.
8. I take care of my body in the best way possible.
9. I am dedicated to taking care of my body.

10. Healthy habits come naturally to me.

11. I am focused on living a healthier life.

12. I am becoming a healthier person every single day.

13. I am learning to make healthier choices.

14. I choose to eat only healthy foods.

15. I am getting healthier thanks to my healthy habits.

16. I take the best care of my body.

17. Healthy habits are easy habits.

18. I am learning more about healthier habits every single day.

19. I rest when my body needs rest.

20. I exercise when my body needs to move.

21. I give my body exactly what it needs to stay healthy.

22. I am always learning how to have healthier habits.

23. I take care of my body with healthy routines.

24. Healthy routines make it easy for me to take care of my body.

25. I create healthy habits and routines that serve my unique needs.

26. I take care of my body the way my body needs me to.

27. I am willing to learn how to take care of my unique body.

28. I always put effort into understanding my body's needs.

29. I educate myself on healthy habits and enforce them as much as I can.

30. I am getting better at maintaining my healthy habits every single day.

31. I fuel my body with healthy habits.

32. I love engaging in healthy habits that make me feel good.

33. My body feels good when I live a healthy life.

34. Healthy habits make me happy.

35. I foster healthier habits in all areas of my life.

36. I adore having a healthier mind, body, and soul.

37. I live to take the best care of myself and my body.

38. I have an easy time fostering new habits.

39. My old habits shed with ease.

40. I pave the way for healthier habits to exist in my life.

41. I am committed to living a healthier, happier life.

42. I choose habits that help me have a higher quality of life.

43. My healthy habits are important to me.

44. I am always making healthier choices.

45. I find it easy to make healthy choices.

46. My quality of life matters, and my healthier habits help me feel better.

47. I love leading a healthy lifestyle.

48. My lifestyle is full of healthy habits.

49. I start my day off with a healthy morning routine.

50. My eating habits are healthy and nutritious.

51. My exercise habits are perfect for my body, my needs, and my goals.

52. I take care of my body in every way that I can.

53. I am always taking care of myself.

54. I have healthy boundaries that serve my healthy lifestyle.

55. I make healthy choices.

56. I always do the best that I can.

57. I find it easy to pick new choices.

58. I release habits that no longer serve me.

59. It is safe to try something newer and healthier.

60. My happiness increases tenfold when I commit to healthier habits.

61. My healthy habits are perfect for my needs.

Affirmations for Self-Esteem

When it comes to body image, self-esteem is important. Low self-esteem can be both the cause of an undesirable body image, and the result of one. If you yourself are unhappy with how you look and feel, it could be because you lack the self-esteem to make a change, or you may feel that way because of how your health is in the present time. Either way, boosting your self-esteem now can help keep you committed to your wellness goals and can improve your ability to foster a body shape and level of health that feels more desirable for you.

1. I deserve a happy, healthy life and body.
2. I am a unique individual.
3. Life is fun and rewarding.
4. I deserve to have a body that helps me explore everything that life has to offer.

5. I choose to be happy and healthy right now. I love my life.

6. I choose to have a healthy experience.

7. I love and accept myself as I am.

8. I am successful now and forevermore.

9. Each day I take a step toward becoming my best self.

10. I deserve to love my body.

11. I am worthy of a positive life experience.

12. I inhale confidence and exhale fear.

13. I am passionate about myself, my life, and my wellbeing.

14. I am a kind and loving person.

15. I am full of energy and enthusiasm.

16. I deserve to take the best care of my body and wellbeing.

17. I am a flexible, adaptable individual.

18. I love thinking positive thoughts about myself and my body.

19. I surround myself with people who love me as I am.

20. My opinions are true to who I am.

21. I surround myself with people who bring out the best in me.

22. I choose to be my best self every single day.

23. I have the power to change myself for the better.

24. I deserve to be loved.

25. I deserve to feel good about myself.

26. I respect myself, my body, and my health deeply.

27. I have something special to offer.

28. I believe in myself.

29. I believe in my ability to achieve my desires.

30. I deserve to feel good about all of me.

31. Improving my self-esteem is important to me.

32. I can feel good about myself while working to better myself every day.

33. I always treat myself and my body with kindness and respect.

34. I am learning to love myself more and more every single day.

35. I choose to love myself.

36. I see myself with kindness.

37. I love myself.

38. I am willing to change to become the best version of me.

39. I approve of myself and my desires.

40. I care about myself, my body, and my wellness.

41. My commitment to myself brings me pleasure.

42. I praise myself freely.

43. I am respected by others as I am.

44. I rejoice in who I am.

45. I deserve to have a great life.

46. I deserve to feel good about my body.

47. I am worthy of wearing clothes that flatter my shape.

48. Each day, I am becoming more confident.

49. I appreciate myself.

50. I appreciate my body.

51. My body loves me.

52. My body deserves to feel good.

53. I nourish myself with healthy thoughts, food, and activities.

54. I care about my wellbeing.

55. I am willing to take better care of myself.

56. I treat my body with the love it deserves.

57. I always choose to love and care for myself.

58. I see my body through the eyes of love.

59. I see myself through the eyes of love.

60. I am willing to fall in love with myself.

61. My body is worthy of feeling it's best.

Affirmations for Beauty

When we are in the process of changing the way our bodies look, it can be difficult to remember that you are beautiful at all stages of your journey, even the parts you don't like. Having affirmations to help you affirm your beauty to yourself will increase your self-esteem, self-confidence, and self-worth while also helping you generally feel better about yourself. Plus, the more beautiful you feel, the more likely you are to invest in your physical wellness and appearance, meaning that you will become even more motivated to nourish yourself well and exercise properly so that you can lose weight *for good*.

1. I am beautiful inside and out.

2. The happier I feel, the more beautiful I become.

3. When I am happy with myself, I am beautiful.

4. My skin is clear, healthy, and glowing.

5. My body is beautiful.

6. I have clean, smooth, and soft skin.

7. I love admiring myself in the mirror.

8. I am a beautiful person.

9. I am grateful for my beautiful body.

10. Each day, my body becomes more beautiful.

11. I am blessed with natural beauty.

12. My body is sexy.

13. I have a healthy, attractive body.

14. Being beautiful comes naturally for me.

15. My body is naturally beautiful.

16. My body shape is flattering.

17. My unique appearance is so beautiful.

18. I have a great sense of style.

19. I present myself with confidence and grace.

20. I am full of health.

21. I am a youthful person.

22. I am comfortable in my own skin.

23. I enjoy being admired by myself and others.

24. I am beautiful as I am.

25. My mind, body, and spirit are beautiful reflections of who I am.

26. I am happy with myself as I am.

27. I radiate true beauty.

28. I choose to laugh and enjoy my life because life is beautiful.

29. The more positive I am, the more beautiful I am.

30. I have beautiful features.

31. Even my flaws are beautiful.

32. My beauty radiates.

33. I take good care of my body and my beauty.

34. I am grateful for being as beautiful as I am.

35. My beauty shines for all to see.

36. I am growing more beautiful every single day.

37. I feel beautiful.

38. My features are growing more attractive every single day.

39. When I take care of myself, my beauty grows.

40. Beauty is a reflection of my inner self-love, and I love myself.

41. I am naturally beautiful.

42. My body has a naturally great shape.

43. The more I take care of myself, the better I look and feel.

44. My entire self is beautiful.

45. People notice how beautiful I am.

46. My beauty is innate.

47. I am uniquely beautiful.

48. I do not compare myself with others. I am beautiful and unique.

49. I see my true beauty.

50. I feel comfortable in my own skin.

51. What I see in the mirror is beautiful.

52. I love my entire self.

53. I see myself as a beautiful, loveable person.

54. I am beautiful.

55. I receive compliments with grace.

56. I deserve to feel beautiful.

57. My inner beauty shows.

58. I am beautiful in all ways.

59. I am a beautiful, radiant person.

60. I welcome my beauty with grace.

61. I choose to feel beautiful.

A Guided Affirmation Meditation

This guided affirmation meditation is an excellent meditation for you to use if you are looking to meditate on something that can improve your mental state and help you feel more positive toward your weight loss goals in general. In this meditation, I have combined a series of positive affirmations that will support you with your weight loss and wellness goals. If you have affirmations that feel more personal and meaningful for you, you can always make your own affirmation meditation with your chosen affirmations. Doing so is a great opportunity to help fill your mind with positive, healthy thoughts and increase your ability to stay positive toward your goals.

This particular affirmation meditation is a short, 10-15-minute meditation. You can do it anytime you need a mental boost. Another great time to use a meditation like this is when you are sleeping, as your brain will be more receptive to what you are listening to while you are sleeping. You can listen to this meditation once through, or listen to the affirmations on repeat as you sleep to help you rewire your subconscious mind and infuse it with the power of these affirmations. What you choose to do and how you choose to use this guided affirmation meditation is entirely up to you and what you feel is going to be most useful in helping you improve your mental state. With that being said, do not use this particular meditation for affirmations when you are driving or doing something that requires your attention as it will help you step into a more relaxed state. If you want something that you can listen to on repeat during the day while you are engaging in other activities, you can create your own audio that consists only of affirmations. Alternatively, YouTube has many great recordings made by people who, like you, want to infuse their minds with positive information that can help them lead lives that make them feel happier and healthier.

The Meditation

To begin this meditation, I want you to start by sitting or lying down in a comfortable place where you can breathe in and out freely. As you do, focus on your breath, and allow yourself to begin to become one with this present moment.

Feel yourself sinking into the present with each breath as you anchor yourself into the here and now. Breathe in, feeling yourself connecting with your body, and breathe out, feeling yourself connecting with this moment. Allow yourself to enjoy the space and freedom of this moment as you indulge in the betterment of yourself and your mind.

As you begin to feel yourself relaxing, I want you to focus even deeper now on your breath. Each time you feel your thoughts being drawn away to something else, gently, and lovingly bring them back to your breath. Feel your chest rising and falling as you breathe in and out. Notice how it feels to have each breath nourish your entire body, mind, and soul with the loving energy of oxygen. Allow yourself to be supported by this natural process as you continue to focus deeply and lovingly on your breath.

While you continue to focus on your breath, I want you to keep an open mind for what is to follow. Feel your mind opening as you breathe in, allowing space for new thoughts that will nurture and support you. Allow any negative or unwanted thoughts to naturally disappear with each exhale. Continue this pattern, now.

In your open mind, repeat after me, while continuing to follow your breathing pattern:

"*I am in control.*

I have the power to decide.

I am in control of my desires.

Self-control comes easily to me.

I can tap into self-control whenever I need to.

I see things through to the end.

I love moving my body.

Today, I will have an excellent workout.

I have a strong body and mind.

My body is becoming healthier every single day.

I am transforming my body every day.

I am losing weight daily.

I am dedicated to taking care of my body.

I choose to eat only healthy foods.

I rest when my body needs rest.

I love leading a healthy lifestyle.

I am always doing the best I can.

I make healthy choices.

I love myself.

I praise myself freely.

I appreciate myself.

I love my body.

I am willing to change to become the best version of myself.

I am a beautiful person.

I treat my body with the respect it deserves.

I am uniquely beautiful.

My beauty is innate.

My entire self is beautiful.

My beauty shines for all to see.

I am naturally beautiful."

As you continue breathing, allow these words to percolate in your mind. Feel them becoming one with who you are, with your identity. Feel yourself affirming that you are, indeed, a strong, capable, beautiful, worthy, and fit human being that can effortlessly lose the weight that you desire to lose. Feel yourself lovingly accepting this new, healthier version of yourself. Allow yourself to become one with this new image of you. Believe the words and affirmations that you have repeated back to yourself and trust that they are true. Commit to believing them.

When you are ready, you can begin to bring your awareness back into the room around you. Allow yourself to open your eyes, return to a natural breathing rhythm, and prepare for the day ahead of you. As you do, feel yourself believing in every single affirmation you heard today, and trusting that it is completely, absolutely true.

Chapter 5: Chakra Guided Meditation

Your seven chakras are located along your spine and represent the seven energetic meridians that connect your body to your spiritual energy. Although they are rooted in spiritual energy and the unseen, your chakras have a huge impact on your physical wellbeing. This includes your ability to create and maintain a healthy body shape and physique. If you want to have your healthiest body in every way possible, you must incorporate spiritual energy work into your practice. This way, you can ensure that you are creating the energetic wellbeing that you need and that you deserve.

In this chapter, we are going to explore what your chakras are, how they affect weight loss, practical steps you can take to nurture your chakras, alternative strategies you can use to heal your chakras, and two important meditations you can use to help your chakras. Our goal here will be to create spiritual wellness within your emotions, mind, body, and soul so that you are able to let go of anything that may be preventing you from losing weight and keeping it off. This will begin to make far more sense as you read through this chapter and understand how these energetic meridians are even affecting you in the first place.

What Are Your Chakras and How Do They Affect Weight Loss?

Your chakras are seven meridians located along your spine. They include your: root, sacral, solar plexus, heart, throat, third eye, and crown chakras. Each chakra represents a certain part of your mental, emotional, physical, and spiritual wellbeing. Ideally, when all of your chakras have been nurtured and balanced, you will find yourself experiencing complete health within your mind, emotions, body, and soul. This means that in addition to feeling grounded and balanced, you will also notice that your physical body actually begins to operate in optimal health. This includes anything and everything relating to your ability to lose weight and create and maintain a healthy and fit body that serves you.

Many cultures and healers, such as hypnosis masters, will tell you that if you focus on the wellbeing of each of your seven chakras, you will have a complete and structured guide for maintaining your wellness overall. They also insist that if you truly want to lose weight and have your healthiest body possible, educating yourself on and taking care of your chakras is crucial to your wellbeing. This is because your chakras are tangible points within your body, but they are also points that represent a bigger picture in your general wellbeing, and in all ways. For weight loss specifically, having healthy chakras means that you are not holding onto anything emotionally, mentally, physically, or spiritually that may be preventing you from having a healthier body. This means that you will release any traumas, negative thoughts, energies, and unhelpful habits or behaviors that may be negatively interrupting your physical wellbeing.

In order to better understand each of your chakras and how they contribute to weight loss and general wellbeing, let's take a brief look at each of your seven chakras.

- **Root Chakra**: Your first chakra is your root chakra, located by the base of your tail bone and represented by the color red. This chakra reflects your physical stability, survival, and instincts. When it is imbalanced, you may retain weight as a way to "guarantee" your survival, sort of like a bear carrying weight to preserve his survival through the winter.

- **Sacral Chakra**: Your second chakra is your sacral chakra, and it is located three finger-widths below your navel. This chakra is represented by the color orange. Carrying some extra weight around your sacral chakra is natural for women of childbearing years, however having too much weight can be unhealthy. Extra weight in this area is often linked to sexual health or sexual trauma.

- **Solar Plexus Chakra**: Your third chakra is your solar plexus chakra, and it is located about three inches above your navel and below your rib cage. It is represented by the color yellow. This chakra represents your feelings of personal power and personal strength. If you have repeatedly had your personal power taken from you or threatened, you may carry extra weight on your body as a way to protect yourself from those who have hurt you in the past. This is often seen as a "barrier" that protects you from the abuse of others. An imbalanced solar plexus chakra does not necessarily mean that you will carry more weight around your mid-section, as this weight may be distributed anywhere across your body.

- **Heart Chakra**: Your fourth chakra is your heart chakra, it is located in the middle of your chest, and it is represented by the color green. Your heart chakra represents your feelings and your emotions. If you are carrying weight due to a lethargic heart chakra, this means that you are carrying emotional burdens that are "too heavy" for you and that need to be released so that you can let go of the extra weight of these burdens.

- **Throat Chakra**: Your fifth chakra is your throat chakra, and it is located at the base of your throat, in that indented space where your throat meets your chest. Your throat chakra is represented by the color blue. Your throat chakra reflects your ability to communicate, including your ability to speak and your ability to hear what others have been saying to you. Your throat chakra may become imbalanced if you are regularly saying unkind things, or if you are regularly hearing unkind things, both of which can lead to you wanting to protect yourself with extra weight to "block" the pain.

- **Third Eye Chakra**: Your third eye chakra is the sixth located between your eyebrows and up about 1-2 finger widths. This chakra is represented by the color indigo. Rarely will an imbalanced third eye chakra lead to weight gain, although an imbalanced third eye can indicate that you are experiencing imbalance elsewhere in your body. Symptoms of imbalance include nightmares, headaches, and struggling to see the entire truth of your life. One way this may translate to wellness could be in your inability to see your own beauty and the reality that you are more than just your body, particularly if you are struggling with body image issues and self-esteem.

- **Crown Chakra**: Located at the crown of your head, directly over your spine, is your seventh chakra. The crown chakra is represented by the color violet. An imbalanced crown chakra means that you are not connected to the divine, which may lead to feelings of loneliness, isolation, or depression, all of which can encourage people to engage in unhealthy behaviors surrounding their wellness.

By balancing each of your seven chakras, you increase your likelihood of being able to effortlessly lose weight in a way that looks and feels good. Through this, you are not only going to create the body image that you want, but you are also going to be able to create the wellness that you desire so that you can genuinely feel happy and healthy in your life. This is imperative when losing weight, as many people do not realize that happiness is not inherently attached to weight loss, but instead to a willingness to accept yourself and respect and support yourself in all ways.

How Integrating Chakra Work Will Help You Lose Weight

Integrating chakra work can help you lose weight by essentially helping you let go of anything that may be preventing you from losing weight, while also fostering habits that help you maintain a healthy weight. Many people find that in choosing to work with their chakras, they discover a healthy and effective structure for how they can approach their wellness as a whole. In order to introduce you to this structure and give you some ideas for how you can integrate your chakras into your wellness and weight loss, let's explore each chakra individually and what you can do to create your desires through that chakra itself.

Your root chakra represents survival and instincts, which means that it connects with your primal subconscious in the deepest way possible. Learning to heal your fears around survival and wellbeing is a great way to allow your instincts to stop instinctively harboring extra weight on your body. This particular symptom often arises when people have grown up in poverty, or in a way that meant they struggled to have access to food or other necessities of survival. Creating a life where you can safely and consistently access healthy food and trusting that your food supply will not run out is a great way to start letting go of habits related to food hoarding and excess eating caused by a fear of survival.

Your sacral chakra represents your sexual urges and energy, as well as your cravings and desires. In order to integrate sacral chakra work into energy loss, you need to balance this chakra so that you can learn how to delay pleasure and desire. This way, you will be less likely to excessively indulge in cravings in order to meet your desires, and when you do choose to mindfully indulge, you will derive far more pleasure from your indulgence. Creating this balance will also help you release any fears you may have around "having enough" and "being enough" so that you can feel more at peace with yourself, your desires, and your desirability.

Your solar plexus chakra represents your personal power and confidence, which is something that many people who are unhappy with their body tend to struggle with. Learning to integrate your solar plexus chakra work by becoming more confident in yourself and more certain in your worthiness is a great way to release any weight or blocked energy that you may be carrying in your solar plexus chakra. As you create this balance, you will find yourself naturally building a body and a life that you feel more comfortable in and confident about.

Your heart chakra represents your emotions, which are something that many people struggle with. Becoming more attuned with your emotions and healing any emotional trauma or pain that you may be carrying is a good way for you to release anything that may be causing you to hold onto weight through your emotions. You will likely find that as you heal, your emotions, energy, and motivation come far more naturally and effortlessly for you.

Your throat chakra represents your ability to communicate and can have a negative impact on your weight when you have been repeatedly told unkind things about yourself, or you have said unkind things about yourself or others on a consistent basis. Learning to have healthier communication and to speak in a more positive and loving tone toward yourself and others is an important step in healing your mindset and laying the foundation for wellness in every way possible. Remember: your mind is the foundation of your entire reality and identity. Healing your communication abilities and habits will help you lay the foundation for healthier communication, a healthier identity, and a healthier reality. You can do this both by changing the way you speak about yourself and others and setting boundaries around how you are willing to allow others to speak about you.

Your third eye chakra can reflect your ability to see the truth and to see the bigger picture. If you want to use your third eye chakra to help you lose weight, you need to be willing to see the truth about yourself and your reality, rather than seeing the narrow view that you may have become obsessed with. Learn how to see the truth in your bigger picture, and how to keep your focus on the end goal. The more you can maintain this focus and vision, the more you will find yourself having better health in your body, mind, emotions, and spirit.

Your crown chakra reflects your ability to remain connected to the divine and to your own divine energy. This divine connection helps you remember that you are not alone, that you are supported, and that you are a valuable and worthy individual. When it comes to weight loss, healing this chakra can help facilitate healing in your lower chakras, such as healing surrounding your survival, desire, cravings, emotions, confidence, and more.

Healing each of your chakras is going to help you clear up any discomfort or dysfunction in your life and spiritual energy that may be leading to you having a difficult time releasing excess weight that you have been carrying. Furthermore, it is going to help you experience more thorough vitality and wellness in your life, making your weight loss about so much more than just weight loss, but also about the creation and integration of a healthier, happier, and more authentic you.

The Seven Chakras and Their Nutritional Guides

Each of the chakras has its own unique guidelines around how you can take care of it. Since we are discussing the topic of weight loss, specifically, let's discuss how you can use each chakra to heal your relationship with food while also nurturing that chakra at the same time. Eating for the wellness of your chakras also happens to be incredibly healing and nurturing to your body, meaning that if you intuitively follow this eating guide or incorporate it into your chosen diet, you will find yourself experiencing greater health overall.

Ideally, you should seek to eat at least one item per chakra per day, although you can look at eating at least one decent serving of each item per week, too. This way, you are more likely to be able to create a healthier diet for yourself while also being able to nurture and care for your body as a whole. If you find yourself struggling to find food sources for each of these particular chakras, you can also use alternative ways to relax and nurture your chakras, which can be found in the next section of this chapter.

For your root chakra, the primary color is red, which means that you want to focus on eating foods that are red. The root chakra also thrives with root vegetables and foods that come out of the ground. Foods like carrots, potatoes, beets, onions, garlic, and radishes are all excellent choices for your root chakra. Protein-rich foods are also ideal, such as eggs, beans, tofu, meats, peanut butter, and soy-based food products. You can also nurture your root chakra using spices such as paprika, chives, and pepper. Eating these foods or even eating a combination of these foods on a routine basis will help nourish your body and keep you healthy, while also helping you maintain a healthy and connected root chakra. Naturally, feel free to adapt your chosen root chakra diet to any diet you may currently be eating to ensure that you are honoring your body and your personal nutritional needs and preferences.

Your sacral chakra is orange, meaning that you want to focus on eating foods that are naturally orange in color. Aside from foods that are orange in color, foods that are naturally sweet or filled with nectar are also great for your sacral chakra. Eat natural raw ingredients like strawberries, mangoes, melons, passion fruit, oranges, and coconut. You can also enjoy raw organic honey, preferably from a local farmer, and various nuts for your sacral chakra. If you want to incorporate spices into your diet to honor your sacral chakra, you can incorporate things like vanilla, cinnamon, and sesame seeds, all of which can be added or infused into various dishes to help you balance your sacral chakra.

Your solar plexus chakra is represented by the color yellow, meaning that you want to eat as much yellow as you can. You can also incorporate citrusy and tropical foods for your solar plexus chakra, as these also carry the energy that nourishes and nurtures this chakra. Eating foods like oats, grains, any variety of rice, flaxseed, and sunflower seeds are all great choices if you want to nurture your solar plexus chakra. You can also eat any variety of dairy products that tend to nurture your solar plexus chakra, such as cheese, milk, yogurt, and milk kefir. If you wish to increase your solar plexus nutritional intake with spices, you can add spices like fennel, turmeric, cumin, chamomile, mint, or ginger to any dish or tea beverage to create a tea that will nurture your solar plexus chakra.

For your heart chakra, you want to focus on eating foods that are naturally green in color. Fortunately, there are many rich green foods that you can enjoy that are known for being highly beneficial to your diet, especially when you are embarking on a weight loss journey. Eating leafy vegetables like kale, spinach, broccoli, dandelion greens, and cabbage are all great vegetables that you can use to help heal and maintain your heart chakra. You can also eat cauliflower, celery, pears, kiwis, and green melons as a way to nourish your heart chakra. For spices, lean toward spices like basil, cilantro, and thyme, all of which are known for nurturing your heart chakra and your actual heart itself, too. If you prefer beverages, incorporate green tea into your daily routine as a way to nurture and nourish your heart chakra.

Your throat chakra is blue, so you want to focus on eating foods that are naturally blue in color. Typically, your throat chakra is more effectively nurtured by liquids such as teas, beverages, syrups, and dressings, all of which are said to be more easily absorbed by the energy of your throat chakra. You can nurture your throat chakra through rich blue fruit juices, such as blueberry juice, mint teas, water, and various herbal teas. Blue pea flower tea is a great option that is known for nurturing your throat chakra, although it may be an acquired taste for some.

Your third eye chakra is indigo, which means you are going to want to nurture this chakra with foods that are indigo in color. Often times, the foods that nurture your throat chakra will also nurture your third eye chakra. For your third eye chakra, focus on eating dark bluish fruits like blackberries, blueberries, and raspberries. You can also enjoy wine or grape juice. Poppy seeds are also said to be highly nutritional and balancing for your third eye chakra.

Your crown chakra is violet, meaning that you need to eat more foods that are violet in color if you want to nurture your crown chakra. Eggplant, purple cauliflower, and purple carrots are great options. Aside from purple foods and drinks, which can sometimes be more challenging to find, you can also enjoy alternative healing and balancing practices that will help you keep your crown chakra in check.

Ideally, you should focus on consuming these foods raw and fresh as often as possible. Of course, that may not always be possible for you, which means that you can opt for getting your servings in through different means, such as frozen or preserved. At the end of the day, making sure that you get these colors and foods in will be more important than anything else, although it is always preferred to opt for natural, organic, and fresh whenever possible. If you do regularly find yourself relying on frozen and preserved goods, you may want to learn how to freeze and preserve the foods yourself so that you can have more control over what is going into your foods. This way, you can avoid excess sugars and unhealthy additives that are often present in frozen or preserved foods that you may get from the store.

Alternatives Ways to Relax and Nurture Your Chakras

Using alternative methods for relaxing and nurturing your chakras is a great opportunity for you to further improve your spiritual wellness while also improving your physical wellness. Most times, alternative methods are known for helping actually improve your physical condition, meaning that things such as your hormones, digestive function, and metabolism will all be improved through maintaining your chakras. In addition to directly impacting your wellbeing, healing your chakras can also help you on a spiritual level, which is said to directly affect your subconscious and further improve your ability to integrate your healing benefits from hypnosis. Most often, those who incorporate both hypnosis and chakra wellbeing into their weight loss journeys experience a form of weight loss that is both rapid and long-lasting.

One way that you can incorporate healing into all of your chakras, while also getting in some exercise and moving your body, is through yoga. Various styles of yoga have been designed to give you the opportunity to move your body and get a proper workout in a while, also healing your chakras. Each pose is meant to help increase your flexibility, open up your energy field, exercise your body, and align your emotions, mind, body, and spirit for a greater sense of wellbeing. You can engage in yoga 3-5 times per week for a great workout that also helps balance your chakras if you are looking for a natural, effective, and nourishing way to balance your chakras.

Other ways to alternatively balance your chakras include meditation, affirmations, incense, crystals, music, and color therapy. Incorporating each of these practices into your chakra healing can help you have more balanced chakras, which will naturally help you shed any stagnant energy that may be causing you to struggle to lose your excess weight. You do not have to engage in every single alternative healing and balancing style to gain benefit from it, however, engaging in one or two is a great way to improve the wellbeing of your chakras and increase your healing capacity so that you can lose weight faster.

For your root chakra, meditating on the space at the base of your spine is a great opportunity to connect with it and help heal it. You can also use affirmations like "I am safe," "I am supported," and "My wellbeing is well cared for." For incense or essential oils, use scents like clary sage, frankincense, cedarwood, rosemary, and rosewood. Crystals like garnet, carnelian, tourmaline, and red jasper are great for your root chakra. You can either keep these crystals nearby or wear them in the form of jewelry as a way to receive the energy that you need from them to aid you in balancing your energy. The root chakra resonates with 396 Hz, so listening to music that has been tuned to 396 Hz from an app like YouTube is a great opportunity to help balance your root chakra through music. For color therapy, wear or surround yourself in things that are red in color to help nurture your energy field with the color red.

Your sacral chakra can be supported by having you meditate on the space below your navel. You can use affirmations like "My life is pleasurable," "I am grateful for the joy of being me," and "I feel completely peaceful from within." Burning incense or using essential oils that have scents like ylang-ylang, rose, clary sage, spearmint, chamomile, eucalyptus, cardamom, or patchouli in them is excellent for helping heal your sacral chakra. If you want to wear crystals or keep them nearby, look into crystals like orange calcite, carnelian, tiger's eye, amber, sunstone, and goldstone. You can listen to music that resonates with 417 Hz if you want to use music to help you heal your sacral chakra. Wearing or surrounding yourself with the color orange is a great way to incorporate sacral chakra healing activities into your life in a subtle yet effective manner.

Your solar plexus chakra can benefit from meditations where you focus on your solar plexus and breathe energy into it. Affirmations like "I am confident and courageous," "I trust in my personal power," and "I am enough," are all great for supporting your solar plexus chakra. If you want to use incense or essential oils, opt for those that have saffron, sandalwood, musk, ginger, or cinnamon in them. Using crystals like citrine, peridot, tiger's eye, amber, and copal are all great for helping you bring gentle healing energy into your solar plexus chakra. Listen to music that resonates with the frequency 528 Hz, which will help activate, awaken, and balance your solar plexus chakra. Surrounding yourself with or wearing the color yellow is a great way to naturally heal your solar plexus chakra.

Your heart chakra can benefit from your using breathing meditations, which will help expand, open, and balance your heart space as well as the energy in your heart chakra. You can use affirmations like "I am worthy of being loved," "I am peaceful," and "I am loving to myself and to others" to help balance your heart chakra. Incense or essential oils that come in scents like orange, sandalwood, jasmine, lavender, and rose are all great scents for your heart chakra. Crystals like peridot, emerald, rose quartz, rhodochrosite, rhodonite, malachite, and aventurine are all great crystals to use to help you heal your heart chakra. Use music that resonates with the frequency of 639 Hz when meditating or doing something relaxing to naturally help soothe and balance your heart chakra. You can also surround yourself in the color green or pink to naturally bring gentle healing energy to your heart chakra.

Your throat chakra benefits from breathing meditations much in the same way that your heart chakra does. As you use a breathing meditation, focus on feeling the air you are breathing in moving through your throat, and expanding and balancing your throat chakra. Use affirmations like "I speak freely and with ease," "I am honest," and "I trust others to allow me to express myself clearly" to help you heal and balance your throat chakra. Using incense or essential oils in scents like jasmine, eucalyptus, cypress, sage, peppermint, geranium, frankincense, tea tree, lavender, and clove are all great for your throat chakra. Crystals such as blue lace agate, blue citrine, turquoise, apatite, azurite, sodalite, and lapis lazuli are all great choices for healing your throat chakra. Listen to music that resonates at the frequency of 741 Hz if you want to use music to gently balance and activate your throat chakra. Wear or surround yourself in bright blues if you want to use color therapy to balance your throat chakra.

Your third eye chakra can benefit from you meditating on the space between and slightly above your eyebrows. You can also use guided visualization meditations as a way to work with, activate, and balance your third eye chakra. Using affirmations like "I see clearly," "I am wise, intuitive, and aligned with my highest good," and "As I tap into my inner wisdom, I know that all is well in my world" is helpful when balancing your third eye chakra. Incenses or essential oils like basil, lemon, jasmine, camphor, frankincense, and myrrh are all great for your third eye chakra. You can also use crystals like amethyst, labradorite, sodalite, lapis lazuli, and purpurite to help you work with balancing your third eye chakra. Listen to frequencies at 852 Hz to help you balance out your third eye chakra if you want to use music therapy, and wear or surround yourself in the color indigo to help you gain access to the healing benefits of color therapy.

For your crown chakra, you can meditate on the space directly above the crown of your head. Simple breathing and mindfulness meditations are great for this space. You can also use affirmations like, "I am one with the Divine," "I know I am safe, loved, and protected," and "I know my higher purpose is being fulfilled now" to help you work with your crown chakra. Incense or essential oils that come in scents like frankincense, camphor, myrrh, and sandalwood are great for your crown chakra. For crystal healing, look at either wearing or surrounding yourself with crystals like amethyst, clear quartz, moonstone, and spirit quartz. Meditate or listen to music at frequencies of 932 Hz for your crown chakra to enjoy sound healing, and surround yourself with the color violet or the color white or any clear objects such as glass decor as a way to instill color healing benefits.

When it comes to healing your chakras, it is important that you approach it from a balanced perspective. Just like with your body: you do not want to emphasize too much on weight loss, desirable appearances, or diet because you will find yourself possibly obsessing in one area and missing the mark in other areas. Instead, focus on creating a well-balanced approach to healing all of your chakras so that you are more likely to experience complete balance overall. You should approach your entire wellness and weight loss journey this way, too, as this will ensure that you are more likely to achieve actual benefits from your journey. This way, you truly feel happy and healthy throughout your journey, and as you achieve your results, rather than feeling as if you have become so fixated on one area of your health that you have forgotten to take care of yourself in other ways.

A Guided Chakra Relaxation Meditation

This simple, guided chakra relaxation meditation is a great meditation that is going to help you bring balance and harmony to your chakras. When it comes to weight loss, creating peace and comfort in your life in all ways as much as possible is a wonderful opportunity to nurture your mind and your body while you work toward making such big changes in your life. Through this, you can balance your hormones and aid your body in naturally adapting to the changes that you are making in such a way that it actually makes it even easier for you to adapt to your healthier lifestyle. Through this, your changes become even easier for you to make, and you are far more likely to maintain these changes in your life.

This meditation should only take about 20 minutes and will help bring great balance and peace to your life. You can do this meditation by either laying down with your spine straight and your legs straight and uncrossed or sitting with your legs crossed and your spine long and tall. If you are sitting, rest your hands on your knees, palm up, so that you can relax and keep your body open and receptive.

The Meditation

When you are ready, begin drawing your awareness into your breath. We are going to take five mindful breaths, breathing in to the count of five and then breathing out to the count of five, as a way to help bring balance and peace to your body. You can start now by focusing on breathing in one, two, three, four, five, and breathing out, one, two, three, four, five. Again, breathe in, one, two, three, four, five, and breathe out, one, two, three, four, five. For the third time, breathe in, one, two, three, four, five, and breathe out, one, two, three, four, five. Fourth breath, breathe in, one, two, three, four, five, and breathe out, one, two, three, four, five. One more time, breathe in, one, two, three, four, five, and breathe out, one, two, three, four, five.

Now, on your next breath in, I want you to visualize sending that breath all the way to the base of your spine where your root chakra is. See your root chakra shining bright red and gently rotating in a clockwise motion like a big red disc at the base of your spine. Visualize your root chakra, receiving the oxygen and energy from your breath, and visualize yourself exhaling any blockages or stagnant energy that may be blocking the flow of your root chakra. Feel yourself breathing into this chakra again as you fuel it with loving energy and feel it balancing and harmonizing in a comfortable and serene manner. As it does, feel your confidence in your stability and your life force growing stronger and deeper.

Now, draw your next breath into your sacral chakra, right below your navel. Feel yourself inhaling life force energy into your navel chakra and exhaling any stagnant energy that may be blocking it from maintaining a harmonized and balanced state. Consciously let go of anything that may be pent up here or causing discomfort in your sacral chakra. See your sacral chakra glowing orange and bright, and getting even brighter every time you inhale and flowing even clearer every time you exhale. Feel it naturally flowing in a gentle clockwise motion, bringing balance and harmony into your energy field. Allow yourself to awaken to a balancing of passion and pleasure as you balance your sacral chakra.

Next, breathe into your solar plexus chakra, between your navel and your rib cage. See this yellow chakra glowing bright and rotating in a clockwise motion as you inhale harmony and balance and exhale stagnant or blocked energy. Continue breathing in deeply and gently as you give yourself plenty of space to bring balance into your solar plexus chakra. Feel yourself growing more confident, self-assured, and courageous with each breath. As you continue breathing, feel your solar plexus chakra growing even more powerful with each breath that you take.

Now, move your breath into your heart space. Feel your chest expanding and opening up to receive energy from each breath, and compressing and releasing any blockages with each exhale. As you do, visualize your heart chakra glowing bright green and rotating clockwise. Feel this chakra growing even more harmonious and balanced with each breath that you take, allowing you to feel your best with each breath that you take. Allow yourself to release any emotional baggage or blockages that you may be carrying, feeling yourself growing more balanced and more peaceful with each breath.

Draw your breath up into your throat space now. Feel your lungs filling and releasing with ease as the air effortlessly passes through your throat and into your lungs. Notice how easily every breath moves through your throat as you breathe, allowing you to feel your best. As you do, see your throat chakra glowing bright blue and gently spinning in a clockwise motion, welcoming balance, and harmony in with ease and grace. Affirm to yourself, "I speak with love," "I communicate with ease," and "I speak my reality into existence." Trust that you are able to create the reality you want through the words you speak and breathe gently with ease and grace.

On your next breath, draw your awareness into your third eye chakra, slightly above and between your eyebrows. Feel your third eye chakra awakening, balancing, and growing more peaceful with every breath you take. Notice the energy in your third eye chakra harmonizing as you watch its indigo color glow bright and see the disc of this chakra rotate gently in a clockwise motion. Feel yourself easing into and enjoying the energy of this chakra with each breath you take. As you breathe in, feel yourself nourishing and balancing this chakra, and when you exhale, feel yourself releasing any blockages that may exist in your third eye chakra.

Lastly, draw your energy and awareness up into your crown chakra. Feel yourself becoming aware of the space directly above your head over your spine. With each breath in, feel your crown chakra becoming more awakened and balanced, and with each breath out, feel yourself releasing any blockages or overwhelm that you may feel within your crown chakra. Allow yourself to feel balanced within your energy as you feel your crown chakra both awakening and spreading gentle harmonizing energy throughout your entire body and all of your lower six chakras.

With all of your chakras balanced and harmonized, spend a few moments focusing on your breath once more. Draw your awareness back into the peaceful and gentle energy of your breath as you once again engage in your five and five breathing session for five breaths. Breathe in for one, two, three, four, five, and breathe out for one, two, three, four, five. Again, breathe in for one, two, three, four, five, and breathe out for one, two, three, four, five. Breathe in, one, two, three, four, five, and breathe out, one, two, three, four, five. Breathe in again, one, two, three, four, five, and breathe out again one, two, three, four, five. One more time, breathe in, one, two, three, four, five, and breathe out, one, two, three, four, five.

Now, let your breath return to a natural and calm state as you allow yourself to meditate in this space of harmony and balance for several moments. Feel yourself feeling completely at peace with yourself and in all areas of your life at this moment. Notice how balanced and comfortable you feel in this space as you allow yourself to experience gratitude for your body at this moment. When you are ready, you can draw your awareness back into the room around you to begin awakening yourself from this meditation. Begin by opening your eyes, then gently shake your body out to awaken yourself from this deep state of meditation. When you feel awakened, you can go about your normal life as you integrate the gentle and meaningful flow of the energy that you have harmonized and balanced here today.

A Guided Chakra Meditation for Healing Your Body Image

Your chakras can go a long way in helping you heal your body image. Through your chakras, you can affirm various aspects of confidence, courage, desirability, and self-worth to yourself. In doing so, you both harmonize and balance your chakras and improve your own connection to yourself and your body image. As you use this meditation, you are going to achieve two important things. First and foremost, you are going to experience a greater sense of balance within each of your chakras that is going to allow you to feel more at peace with your body. This is going to allow you to love and respect your body at all stages of your journey, even the ones where you may not be particularly happy with your body or where you may want to change your body.

Next, you are going to experience a sense of balance in areas where you cannot change your body and where no amount of exercising or dietary practices will change anything for you. Sometimes, there are parts of our bodies that we cannot change, and we simply have to learn how to love and accept them, even if we are not particularly fond of them. This does not necessarily mean that you have to like this part of your body, but it does mean that it is a good idea for you to stop hating this part of your body so that you can find peace and acceptance in it instead.

For this meditation, you will need about 15-20 minutes, and you can complete it either while lying down or while sitting with your legs crossed and your spine straight. If you choose to sit up, keep your hands on your knees, palms up, and keep your body engaged and activated. This way, you are balancing your chakras simply from holding this healthy and aligned posture.

The Meditation

Begin this meditation by taking a nice deep breath in, slowly filling up your lungs with fresh, nourishing oxygen, and then exhaling it slowly. Breathe as slowly as you can, feeling each breath getting slower and slower as you gently fill your lungs up with oxygen and then release that oxygen from your lungs once again. Allow yourself to naturally lengthen and slow down each breath so that you can feel yourself deeply relaxing. As each breath grows longer and slower, you will feel yourself naturally sinking into a deeper and more relaxed state. With each breath, feel your relaxation and peace doubling as you allow yourself to completely embrace yourself with calm, gentle energy.

If you find your mind wandering as you work towards this relaxed state, allow yourself to gently draw your awareness back to your breath. Use the consistent and gentle flow of energy moving in and out of your lungs as a rhythm to keep your awareness focused and intentional. Take care to keep yourself as still, mindful, and engaged as possible while also allowing your conscious mind and body to relax completely.

When you are ready, send your awareness down to your root chakra. See it glowing bright red and flowing in a clockwise motion. As you keep your awareness in your root chakra, see yourself becoming aware of all of the body parts associated with your root chakra, including your: legs, feet, glutes, and bones. Allow yourself to lovingly send energy to each of these parts of your body as you mindfully accept them and express gratitude for them and all that they do for you. Send love to your legs and feet for holding you up and assisting you with walking or moving through life in a meaningful manner. Send love to your glutes for giving you a comfortable seat, and to your bones for holding your body together and upright. If you have any flaws within any of these areas of your body, send love to these flaws and accept them as they are. Accept yourself as you are.

Now, send your awareness up into your sacral chakra. See your sacral chakra glowing bright orange and gently flowing in a clockwise motion. As your awareness grows more attached to this part of your body, consider the parts of your body that your sacral chakra governs. Think about your sexual organs and your perception of your own attractiveness. Think about your adrenal glands, kidneys, and even your bladder. Send love and gratitude to each of the body parts that your sacral chakra governs. Accept these parts of your body as they are, and thank them for all of the work they do in helping you maintain a high quality of life. Think about the parts that you can see and interact with, such as your sexual attraction. Send thanks to your body for being attractive, and gratitude for your ability to increase your attraction. Affirm your attractiveness and express gratitude for your increasing attraction. See yourself as having the attractive body that you desire, and see yourself as being desired by others for your attractive body, too.

Next, draw your awareness into your solar plexus chakra. Feel your solar plexus chakra glowing bright yellow and rotating in a gentle clockwise motion as you draw your awareness into this part of your body. Become aware of the parts of your body that your solar plexus chakra governs, such as your stomach, your digestive organs, and your diaphragm. Send gratitude to your solar plexus chakra for all that it offers you in life, and send love and acceptance to the parts of your body that it governs. Ask for forgiveness for always fixating on the extra weight that it carries and invite it to release that weight naturally and rapidly as you commit to loving and accepting yourself as you are. Visualize the weight naturally dropping off and your stomach taking on the shape that you have always desired.

Draw your awareness up now into your heart chakra, feeling it glowing bright green and rotating gently in a clockwise motion. Draw your awareness into your heart chakra and all parts of your body that are governed by your heart chakra, including your chest, your lungs, and your circulatory system.

See yourself as having a desirable and attractive chest, strong muscles, and a healthy circulatory system. Feel your stamina increasing with each breath, and see yourself as having the level of fitness that you desire. Send love, gratitude, and acceptance to your heart chakra for all that it does for you, and to all of those parts of your body and how they support you in experiencing your best possible life.

Now, draw your awareness up into your throat chakra. See your throat chakra glowing bright blue and gently rotating in a clockwise motion. As you do, allow yourself to become aware of the parts of your body that your throat governs, including your neck, your ears, and your respiratory system. Send gratitude and love to the unseen parts of life that your throat chakra governs. Accept your throat chakra as it is, and visualize it naturally slimming as your throat and neck become shapelier and even more attractive. Appreciate your throat and neck for how they look now and for how they have served you all of your life.

Again, draw your awareness up and into your third eye chakra. See your third eye chakra glowing bright indigo and gently spinning in a clockwise motion. Allow yourself to become aware of the parts of your body that your third eye chakra govern, including your mind and your face. Feel yourself sending love and gratitude to your mind and accepting yourself for the beautiful and unique individual that you are. Allow yourself to accept and love your face and all of your facial features and the way they help you look unique and attractive. Send gratitude to your face for your ability to slim your body down and see beauty in your reflection every time you look in the mirror. Appreciate yourself for who you are, and for who you are becoming every single day.

Lastly, draw your awareness up into your crown chakra. See your crown chakra glowing bright violet and gently rotating clockwise. Become aware of your entire self and all that makes you, you, and send love, gratitude, and acceptance to yourself. Become willing to fall in love with yourself as you are, and feel how deeply connected you feel with yourself and all of life that surrounds you when you embrace this deep level of connection and love. Feel how peaceful and meaningful this is for you to fall into such a deep level of love and acceptance with yourself, including all that you can and cannot change, and all that you do and do not like about yourself. Understand that no matter what, you can choose to love yourself, even if you do not like everything about yourself.

Spend a few moments in this space, breathing and meditating into these feelings of love, acceptance, and gratitude that you are now feeling for yourself and your body. Then, when you are ready, awaken yourself by opening your eyes and gently shaking your limbs out so that you can bring energy and awareness back into the present moment. Allow yourself to approach the rest of the day and every day from here on out with great love, gratitude, and acceptance for yourself and trust that you can love yourself both now and later when you have achieved your ideal body image. From this place of love, acceptance, and gratitude, you will be far more likely to achieve your goals and feel truly happy and healthy in your new slimmer and stronger body.

Conclusion

Losing weight is a journey that is not always easy. Often times, people think it is as simple as changing your diet and including some exercise in your daily routine and just like that everything changes. While diet and exercise are undeniably important aspects of weight loss, focusing exclusively on diet and exercise means that you are forgetting one important thing: your mind. Your mind is responsible for all of the habits and behaviors you engage in, including the ones that lead to you relying on an unhealthy diet and unhealthy exercise routine in the first place. If you truly want to lose weight and keep the weight off, you need to take your mind, emotions, and spirit into account, too.

I hope that after reading *Extreme Weight Loss Hypnosis,* you have a deeper understanding of the importance of your mind and how you can incorporate it into your weight loss journey. Through proper hypnosis practices, mindset shifts, and energy practices, you can help rewire your brain so that embracing healthier habits and behaviors comes easily for you. This way, rather than struggling and fighting against your inner voice, which is asking you to behave in one way (an unhealthy way), you can flow naturally with your body and inner voice into a state of better health.

After you finish reading this book, I encourage you to maintain a journal and continue to document your journey. Pay attention to what meditations you are using, how they make you feel, and what you are gaining from each session. Also, pay close attention to your habits and behaviors, including the mindset and thoughts that drive them. The more honest you can be with yourself, the better, as this honesty will allow you to shed light on what is actually affecting you in your life and what you can do about it.

Remember that weight loss is a journey and not a sprint, so take your time and be consistent in your practice. The more consistent you are with your mindset, diet, and exercise, the faster you are going to see your weight shedding. If you truly want to go fast, be consistent, and stay focused on mastering each step with excellence.

Before you go, I ask that you please take a moment to review *Extreme Weight Loss Hypnosis* on Amazon Kindle. Your honest feedback on this book would be greatly appreciated, as it helps me understand what you want and need so that I can create even more great content for you going forward.

Thank you, and remember that this journey is not as challenging as you think. You can make it easier for yourself, and you can absolutely have control over your ability to enjoy a happier and healthier body. Stay focused, and trust in yourself!

CPSIA information can be obtained
at www.ICGtesting.com
Printed in the USA
LVHW010942210121
676969LV00001B/61